From Microbes to Medicines: Harnessing the Power of Immunity

OrangeBooks Publication

1st Floor, Rajhans Arcade, Mall Road, Kohka, Bhilai, Chhattisgarh 490020

Website: **www.orangebooks.in**

First Edition, 2025

ISBN: 978-93-7426-692-2

Price: Rs. 310.00

Printed in India

FROM MICROBES TO MEDICINES

HARNESSING THE POWER OF IMMUNITY

NITYA BYRRAJU

OrangeBooks Publication
www.orangebooks.in

Contents

Part I: The Invisible World

Understanding the Tiny Life Forms that Surround us Every Day

Chapter - 1
Meet Your Microscopic Neighbours

"The tiny living things all around us"

The Invisible World Around Us

Imagine a world so small that millions of living creatures could fit on the tip of a needle. This invisible world exists all around us, on us, and even inside us. These tiny life forms are called microbes, and they are everywhere - in the air we breathe, the water we drink, the soil we walk on, and throughout our bodies.

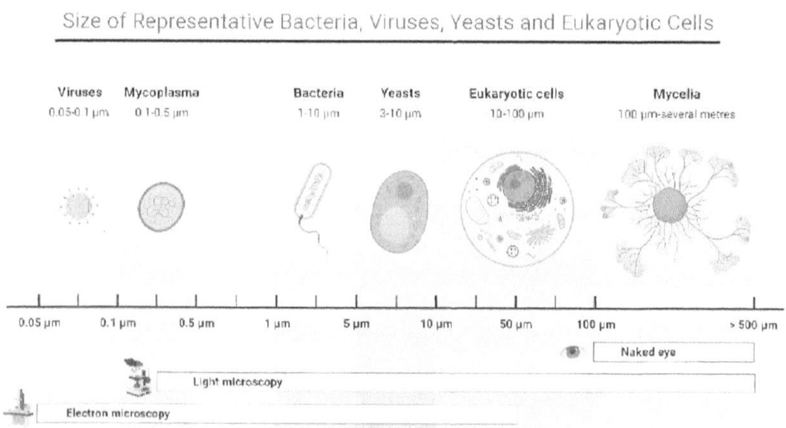

Pic 1: https://microbeonline.com/size-of-bacteria/

Microbes are so small that we need special instruments called microscopes to see them. To understand just how tiny they are, think of it this way: if a microbe were the size of a marble, then a marble would be the size of the Earth. That's how incredibly small these creatures are, yet they play enormous roles in our daily lives.

What Are Microbes? Understanding the Four Main Types

There are four main types of microbes that affect human health. Bacteria are single-celled organisms that look like tiny rods, spheres, or spirals under a microscope. Many bacteria are actually helpful to us. They live in our intestines and help us digest food, they make yogurt and cheese taste good, and they even help plants grow by adding nutrients to soil.

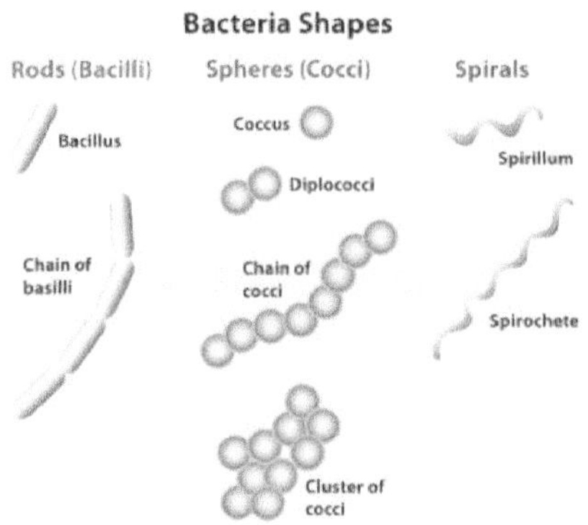

Pic 2: https://www.dreamstime.com/

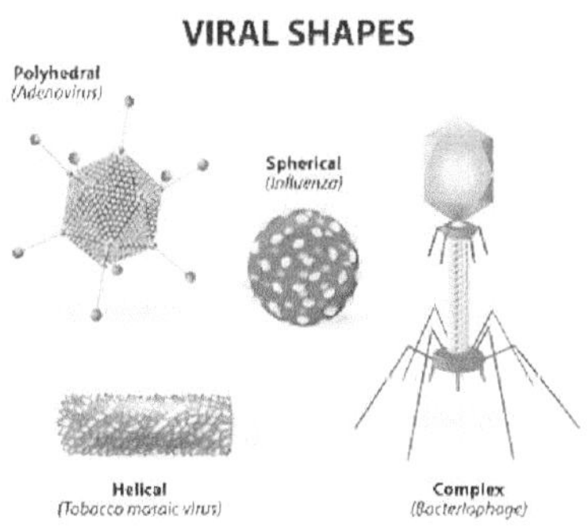

Pic 3: https://www.shutterstock.com/

Viruses are even smaller than bacteria and are quite different. While bacteria can live and reproduce on their own, viruses need to get inside other living cells to survive and multiply. Think of viruses as tiny pirates that hijack our body's cells to make copies of themselves. Common cold and flu are caused by viruses.

Fungi include things like mushrooms that we can see, but also tiny yeasts and molds that we cannot see without a microscope. Some fungi help make bread rise and give cheese its flavor, while others can cause infections on our skin or in our lungs, especially in damp conditions.

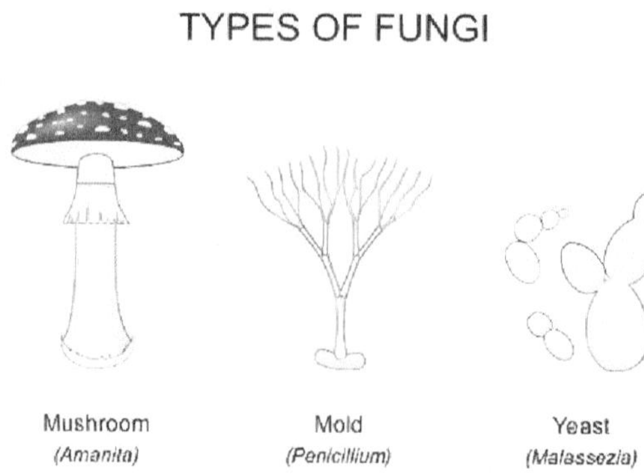

Pic 4: https://www.dreamstime.com/

Types of Parasites

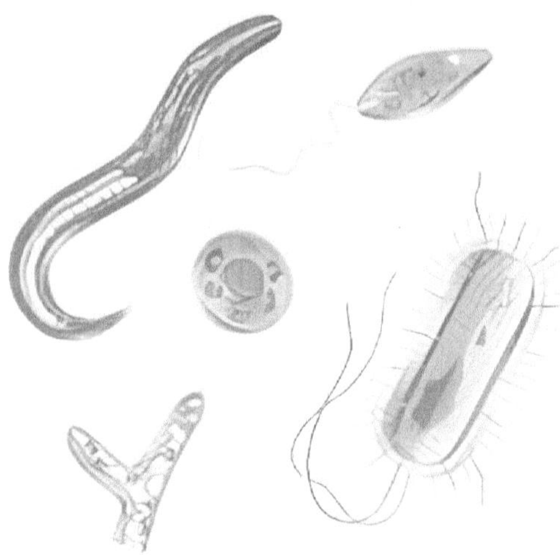

Pic 5: https://www.safewater.org/

Parasites are microbes that live by taking what they need from other living things. They include tiny worms, single-celled organisms, and other creatures that can make us sick by living inside our bodies and taking our nutrients.

Good Microbes vs. Harmful Ones

Most microbes around us are either helpful or harmless. In fact, our bodies contain roughly the same number of helpful bacteria as we have human cells. These good bacteria help protect us from harmful ones, help us digest food, and even help make some vitamins our bodies need.

The harmful microbes, often called germs or pathogens, are actually in the minority. However, when these bad microbes get into our bodies in large numbers or when our body's defenses are weak, they can cause infections and make us sick.

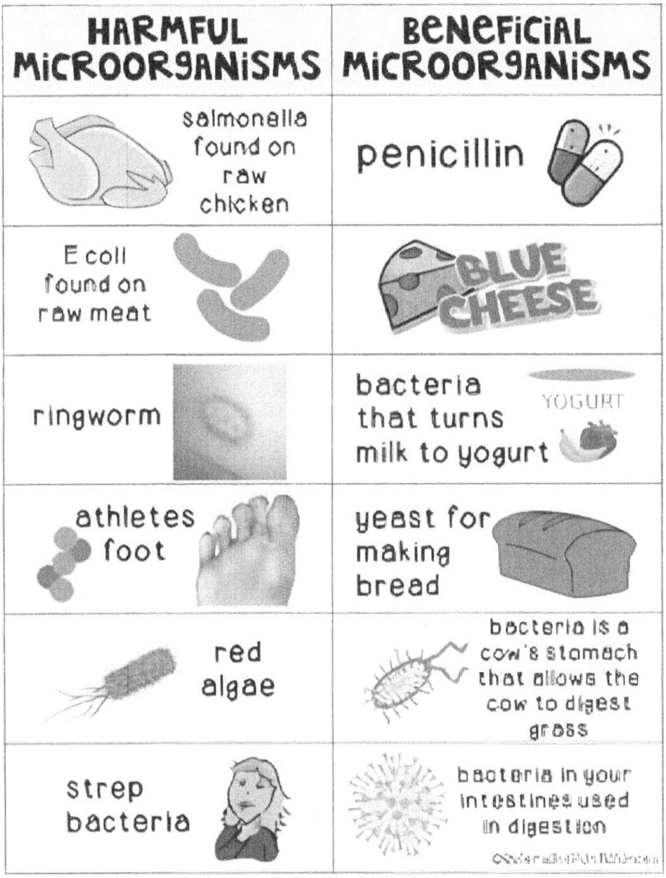

Pic 6: https://in.pinterest.com/pin/344032859036456828/visual-search/

Where Microbes Live: In Our Bodies, Water, Soil, and Air

Understanding microbes helps us make better decisions about staying healthy. When we know that most microbes are harmless and that our bodies are designed to handle them, we can focus our energy on the practices that really matter for preventing illness.

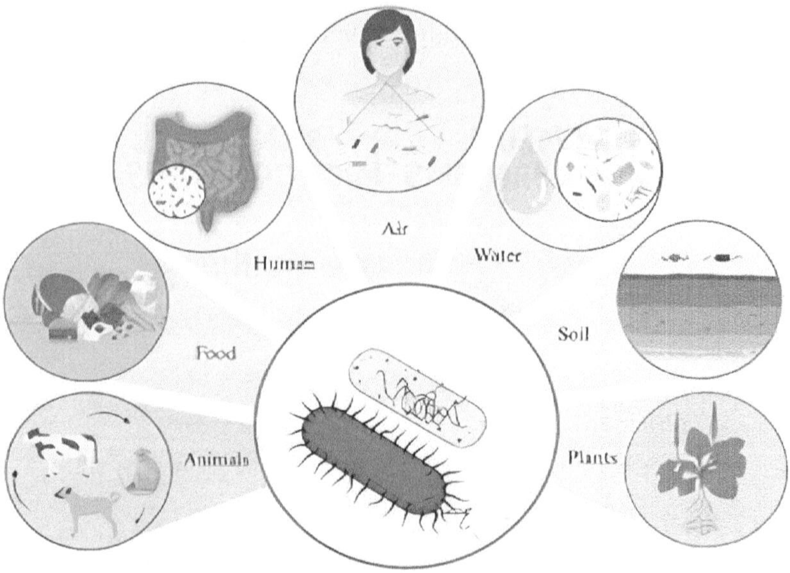

Pic 7: https://www.frontiersin.org/

Community Focus: Microbes in Crowded Living Conditions

In crowded living conditions, microbes spread more easily between people. When many people share small spaces, use the same water sources, or have limited access to clean bathrooms, harmful microbes can pass from person to person more quickly. This doesn't mean that people in these conditions are dirty or bad-it simply means that microbes have more opportunities to travel.

Chapter - 2
How Infections Happen

"When unwanted guests move in"

Understanding Infection: When Harmful Microbes Move In

An infection occurs when harmful microbes enter our body, find a place to live, and begin to multiply. It's like having uninvited guests who not only enter your home but also invite all their friends to move in with them. Understanding how these unwanted guests get inside helps us know how to keep them out.

How Germs Enter Our Body: The Main Entry Points

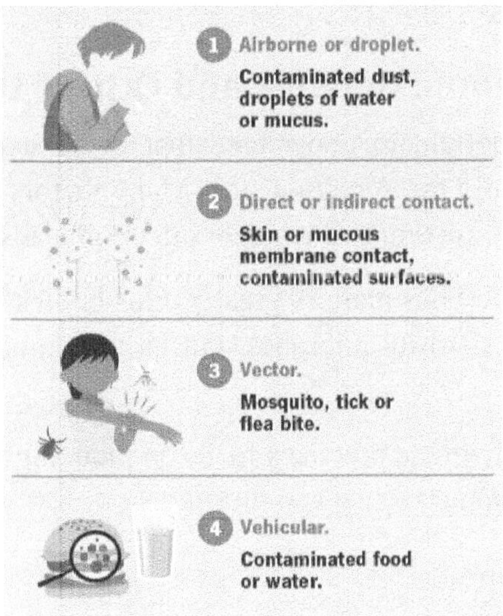

Pic 8: https://my.clevelandclinic.org/

Microbes have several main doorways into our bodies. Our skin is usually an excellent barrier, but any break in the skin - from a small cut, scrape, or insect bite-can become an entry point. This is why cleaning wounds properly is so important, even tiny ones.

We also breathe in microbes from the air around us. When someone with a respiratory infection coughs or sneezes, they release thousands of tiny droplets containing microbes into the air. If we breathe in these droplets or they land on surfaces we touch, the microbes can enter through our nose, mouth, or eyes.

Our digestive system is another common entry route. Microbes can enter through contaminated food or water. This happens when food is not cooked properly, when water sources are contaminated with sewage, or when hands are not washed before eating. The microbes then travel down to our stomach and intestines, where they may cause illness.

Insects like mosquitoes, flies, and ticks can also carry microbes from one person to another or from animals to people. When these insects bite, they can inject microbes directly into our bloodstream. Mosquitoes, for example, can transmit malaria parasites, while flies can carry bacteria from waste to food.

Why Some People Get Sick and Others Don't

However, it's important to understand that being exposed to microbes doesn't automatically mean getting sick. Many factors determine whether exposure leads to infection and whether infection leads to illness.

The number of microbes matters greatly. Our bodies can usually handle small numbers of harmful microbes, but large numbers can overwhelm our defenses.

This is why good hygiene practices focus on reducing the total number of microbes we encounter.

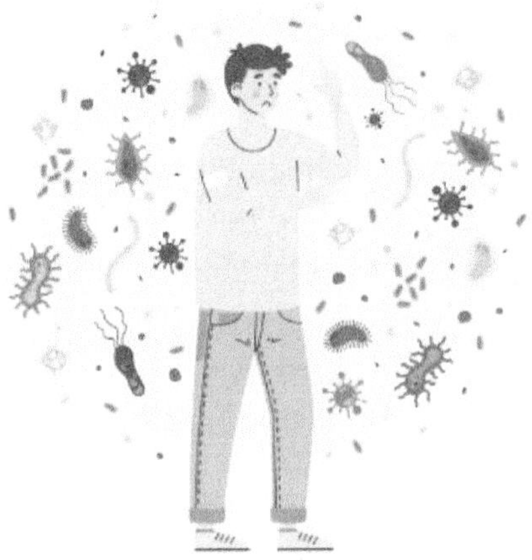

Pic 9: https://www.freepik.com/

The strength of our immune system also plays a crucial role. People who are well-nourished, get enough sleep, and aren't under extreme stress usually fight off infections better than those whose immune systems are weakened.

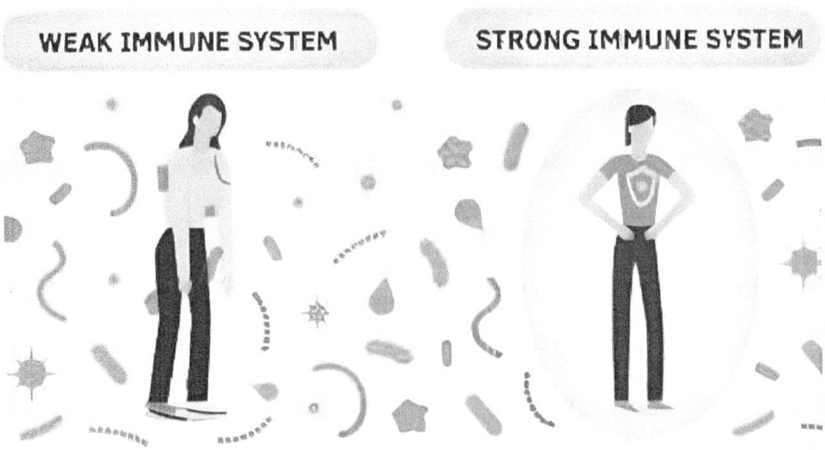

Pic 10: https://www.shutterstock.com/

Some people have natural resistance to certain infections due to their genetics or previous exposure. Others may be more susceptible because of age, underlying health conditions, or malnutrition.

The Difference Between Being Infected and Being Sick

Understanding these pathways helps explain why some infections spread quickly through communities while others remain isolated cases. It also helps us understand that preventing infection often requires community-wide solutions, not just individual actions.

Community Focus: Common Infection Routes in Slum Environments

In crowded living conditions, infections can spread more easily for several reasons. When many people share small spaces, there are more opportunities for microbes to pass from person to person through breathing, touching, or sharing items. Limited access to clean water makes it harder to maintain good hygiene practices that prevent infection.

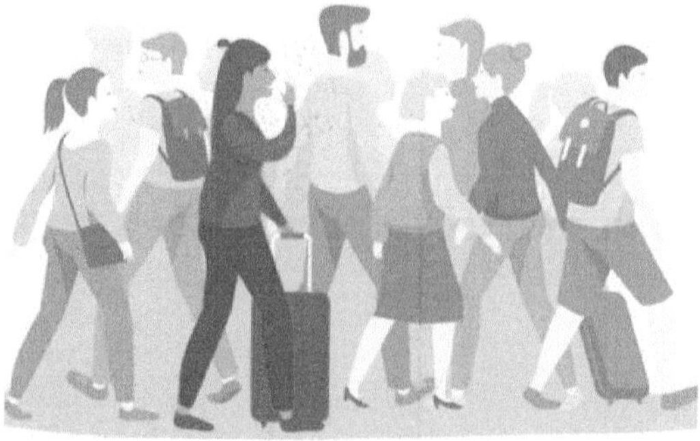

Pic 11: https://www.shutterstock.com/

Shared cooking and eating spaces can allow contaminated food or water to affect many people at once. When bathroom facilities are shared or inadequate, microbes from human waste can more easily contaminate water sources or living areas.

Poor drainage and waste management can create breeding grounds for insects that carry disease. Standing water provides places for mosquitoes to lay eggs, while improperly disposed waste attracts flies.

Chapter - 3
Your Body's Defense Army

"How your body fights back"

Simple Explanation of the Immune System

Your body has an amazing defense system that works day and night to protect you from harmful microbes. This system, called the immune system, is like having a well-trained army with different types of soldiers, each with special jobs to keep you healthy.

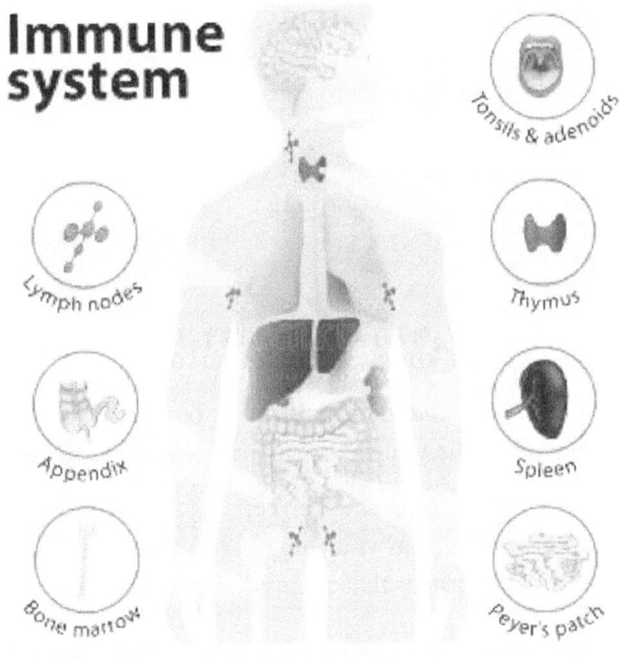

Pic 12: https://www.dreamstime.com/

The First Line of Defense: Your Body's Barriers

The first line of defense starts with barriers that keep microbes from entering your body. Your skin acts like a strong wall around a castle. It's slightly acidic, which makes it harder for many harmful microbes to survive on its surface. Your skin also constantly sheds old cells, taking away any microbes that might be trying to establish themselves.

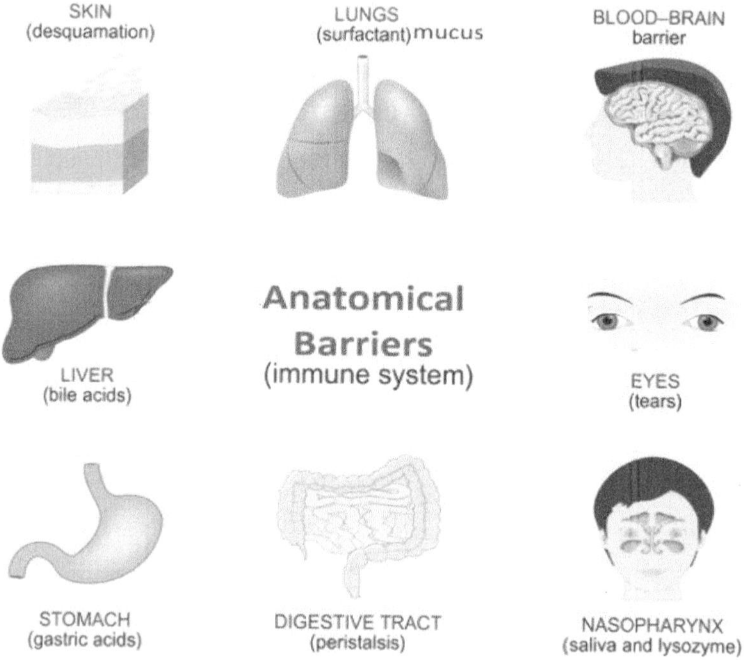

Pic 13: https://www.shutterstock.com/

Inside your body, you have other protective barriers. The mucus in your nose and throat traps microbes like flypaper catches flies.

Tiny hairs called cilia constantly sweep this mucus upward, carrying trapped microbes away from your lungs. Your stomach produces strong acid that kills most microbes that enter with food or water.

White Blood Cells as Soldiers

When microbes do manage to get past these barriers, your immune system's mobile defense force springs into action. White blood cells are the soldiers of this army, and there are several different types, each with special abilities.

Some white blood cells act like guards on patrol. They constantly circulate through your body looking for anything that doesn't belong. When they find harmful microbes, they can either eat them directly or call for help from other immune cells.

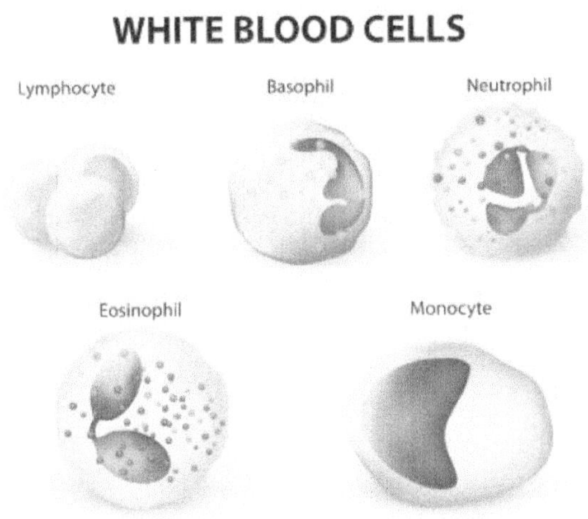

Pic 14: https://www.dreamstime.com/

Other white blood cells are like specialized soldiers trained to fight specific enemies. Once your body encounters a particular type of microbe, these cells remember it. If the same microbe tries to invade again, these memory cells can quickly organize a defense, often preventing you from getting sick at all.

How Fever, Swelling, and Pain Actually Help

When your immune system is fighting an infection, you may notice several changes in your body. Fever is one of the most common signs. While fever makes you feel uncomfortable, it's actually helping your body fight infection. Most harmful microbes grow best at normal body temperature, so raising your temperature makes it harder for them to multiply. Fever also helps your immune cells work more effectively.

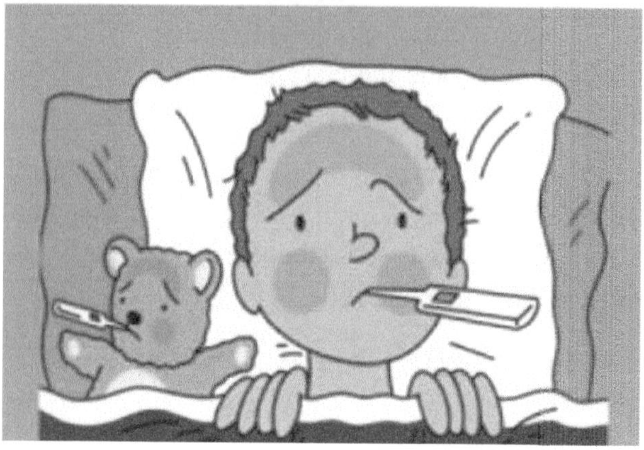

Pic 15: https://annapolispediatrics.com/

Swelling and redness around cuts or infected areas show that your immune system is sending extra blood and immune cells to fight the infection. The increased blood flow brings more soldier cells to the battle and helps carry away waste products from the fight.

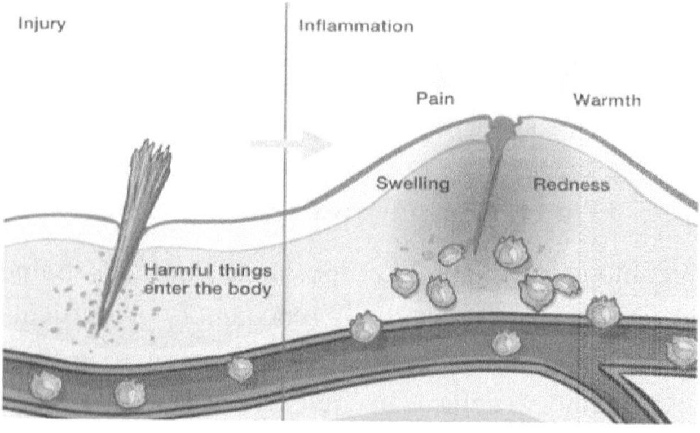

Pic 16: https://www.aboutkidshealth.ca/

Pain can also be part of your body's defense strategy. Pain makes you want to rest the affected area, which helps your body focus energy on healing rather than on other activities.

Why Rest and Nutrition Matter for Immunity

Your body's ability to fight infection depends heavily on having the right raw materials. Good nutrition provides the building blocks your immune system needs to make new white blood cells and antibodies. Protein is especially important because immune cells are made largely of protein.

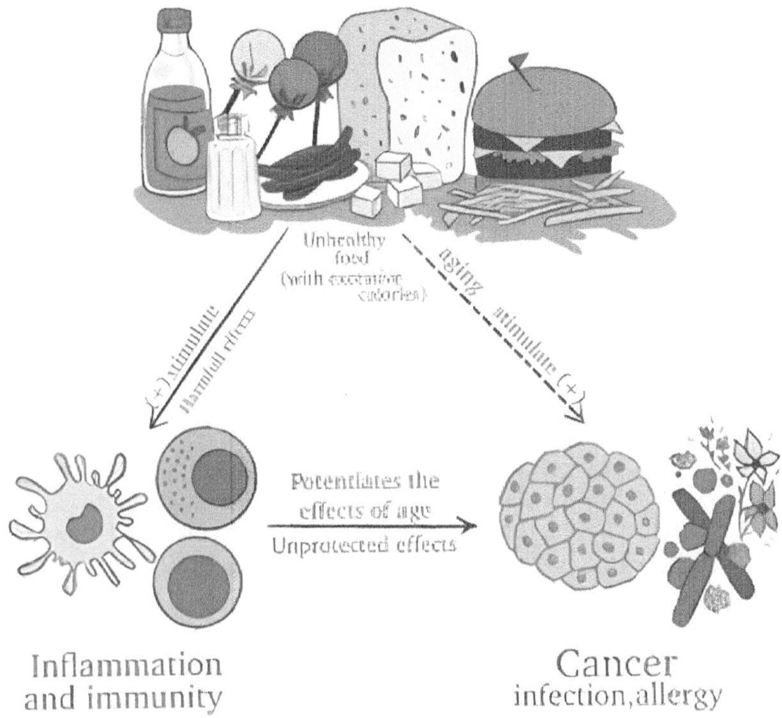

Pic 17: ttps://www.frontiersin.org/

Sleep is crucial for immune function. During sleep, your body produces more infection-fighting cells and antibodies. People who don't get enough sleep are more likely to get sick when exposed to viruses.

Stress can weaken your immune system. When you're constantly worried or anxious, your body produces hormones that can suppress immune function. This is why people often get sick during particularly stressful periods.

Community Focus: Strengthening Immunity with Limited Resources

In communities with limited resources, supporting immune function requires creativity and community cooperation. Sharing nutritious foods when possible helps ensure everyone gets some variety in their diet. Beans, lentils, and other legumes provide protein even when meat is expensive. Green leafy vegetables, even those that grow wild, contain vitamins that support immune function.

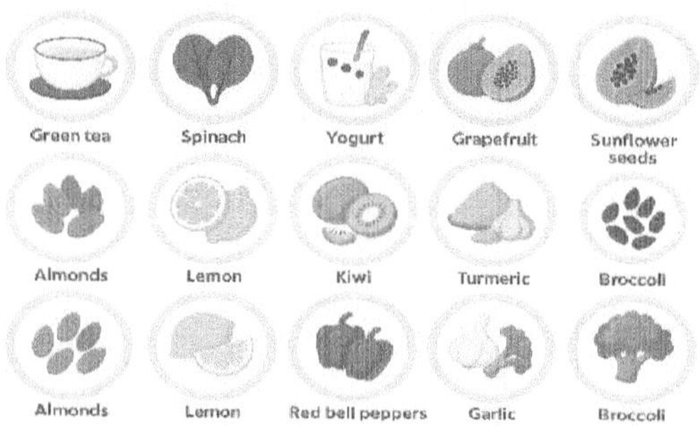

Pic 18: https://www.shutterstock.com/

Creating opportunities for adequate rest, even in crowded conditions, helps everyone stay healthier. This might mean establishing quiet times when children can nap or taking turns so that sick family members can rest undisturbed.

Managing stress through community support, shared childcare, or simply having someone to talk to about problems can help maintain immune function during difficult times.

Traditional remedies that have been used for generations often support the immune system even if they don't directly kill microbes. Ginger, turmeric, and other spices have properties that can help reduce inflammation and support healing.

Understanding how your immune system works helps you make choices that support your body's natural ability to fight infection. It also helps you understand when your body needs extra help and when to seek medical care.

Chapter - 4

Reading the Signs - When Your Body Tells You Something's Wrong

"Learning to listen to your body's warnings"

Understanding Your Body's Alarm System

Your body has an excellent communication system that sends you messages when something isn't right. Learning to understand these signals can help you take care of minor problems before they become serious and know when you need to seek help from others.

Every person's body has its own normal patterns. Some people naturally run a little warmer or cooler than others. Some have more energy in the morning, while others feel best in the evening. Learning your own normal patterns helps you recognize when something is changing.

Common Warning Signals: Fever, Fatigue, Pain, and Changes in Breathing or Eating

Changes in energy levels often signal that your body is working hard to fight infection. Feeling more tired than usual is your body's way of telling you to rest so it can focus energy on healing. Suddenly feeling much more tired, especially with other symptoms, can indicate that an infection is getting worse.

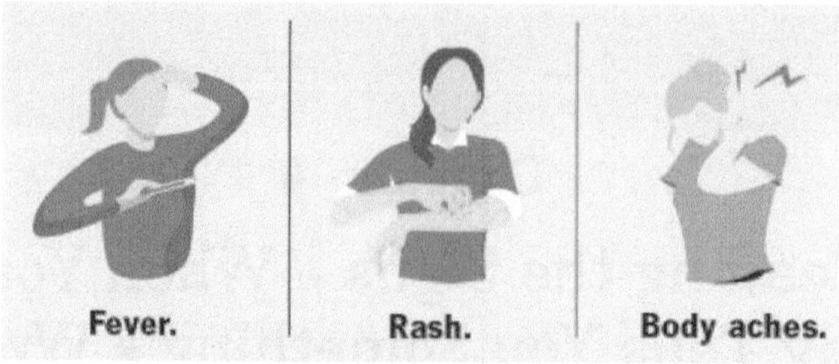

Pic 19: https://my.clevelandclinic.org/

Changes in appetite often accompany infections. While loss of appetite is common when fighting infection, being unable to keep down fluids for more than a day or two is a warning sign that needs attention. In children, refusing to drink fluids is particularly concerning.

Pain serves as an important warning system. New pain that gets progressively worse over hours or days often indicates that something needs attention. Sharp, severe pain that comes on suddenly is usually more concerning than mild, constant discomfort.

Changes in breathing patterns can indicate respiratory infections or other serious problems. Breathing that becomes noticeably faster, more difficult, or makes unusual sounds needs prompt evaluation. In children, pulling in of the skin around the ribs when breathing indicates difficulty.

Skin changes can also provide important clues. A rash that appears along with fever might indicate a specific type of infection. Skin that becomes very pale, bluish, or develops red streaks needs immediate attention.

Fever Patterns and What They Mean

Fever is one of the most important signals to understand. A mild fever in adults - between 100 and 102 degrees Fahrenheit - usually means your body is fighting an infection and is often not dangerous by itself. However, the pattern of fever can tell you important information about what's happening.

A fever that comes and goes might indicate a different type of infection than a fever that stays constant. Fevers that are higher at night and lower in the morning are common with many infections. A fever that rises very quickly or goes very high needs immediate attention.

In children, fever patterns can be different from adults. Children can develop high fevers quickly with infections that would cause only mild fever in adults. However, children also recover from fevers more quickly once their bodies fight off the infection.

Community Patterns: When Infections Spread

Understanding when many people in a community get similar symptoms helps identify outbreaks that might need coordinated response. When several people develop diarrhea at the same time, it often indicates contaminated water or food. Respiratory symptoms affecting many people might mean a contagious virus is spreading.

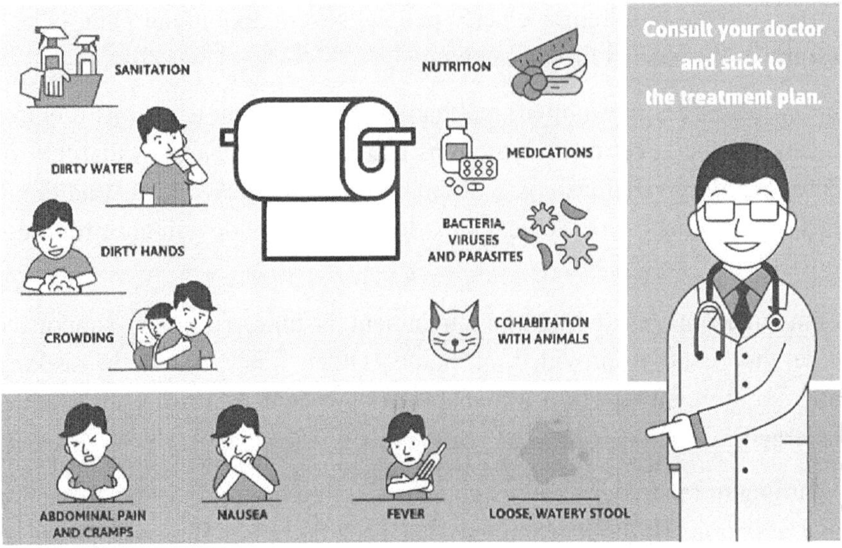

Pic 20: https://www.vukuzenzele.gov.za/

Seasonal patterns help predict and prepare for certain infections. In many areas, respiratory infections are more common during cooler months when people spend more time in crowded indoor spaces. Diarrheal diseases often increase during hot seasons when food spoils more quickly and flies are more active.

Environmental clues from your living situation can help explain why infections occur and how to prevent them. Standing water around homes provides breeding places for mosquitoes. Improperly stored food attracts flies and rodents that can spread disease. Overcrowded sleeping areas make respiratory infections spread more easily.

Making Smart Healthcare Decisions

Deciding when you can manage symptoms at home and when you need outside help is a crucial skill. Mild symptoms that improve gradually over a few days usually don't require immediate medical attention. However, symptoms that get progressively worse over 24-48 hours often need evaluation.

Certain warning signs should never be ignored, regardless of other factors. These include difficulty breathing, severe dehydration, high fever in very young children or elderly people, severe abdominal pain, or any symptom that seems life-threatening.

When resources are limited, making smart healthcare decisions requires balancing the severity of symptoms against the cost and availability of care. Building relationships with community health workers, traditional healers, or others with medical knowledge can provide guidance for these difficult decisions.

Sometimes the most important treatment is time, rest, and supportive care that can be provided at home. Other times, delay in seeking appropriate care can turn a manageable problem into a life-threatening emergency.

Learning to read your body's signals is a skill that improves with practice and attention. By understanding what your body is telling you, you can take better care of yourself and your family, make informed decisions about when to seek help, and often prevent minor problems from becoming major ones.

The key is learning to listen carefully to what your body is saying, understanding which signals are urgent and which are not, and knowing what resources are available in your community when you need help beyond what you can provide at home.

Part II: Knowing Your Enemy

Understanding the Different Types of Germs That Can Make Us Sick

Chapter - 5
Bacterial Infections - The Single-Cell Invaders

"Understanding bacteria and what they do"

What Are Bacteria?

Size and Appearance - Single Cells That Multiply Fast

Bacteria are among the simplest forms of life on Earth, yet they are incredibly successful at survival and reproduction. Each bacterium is made up of just one cell, but don't let this simplicity fool you. These single cells are like tiny, efficient factories that can do everything needed to stay alive and make copies of themselves.

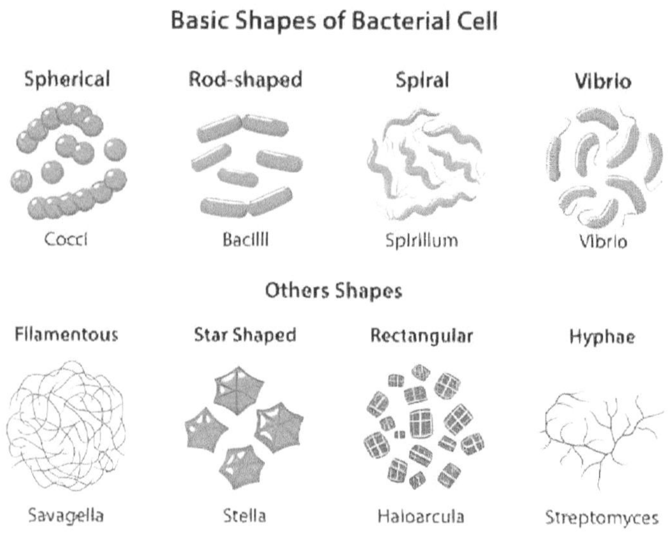

Pic 21: https://www.shutterstock.com/

To understand how small bacteria are, imagine trying to line them up side by side. You could fit about 1,000 bacteria across the width of a single human hair. Even though they're invisible to our naked eyes, bacteria come in several distinct shapes that scientists use to identify them.

Some bacteria look like tiny rods or sticks under a microscope. These rod-shaped bacteria are called bacilli, and they include the bacteria that cause tuberculosis and many types of food poisoning. Other bacteria are perfectly round, like microscopic balls. These sphere-shaped bacteria are called cocci, and they include the bacteria that cause strep throat and some types of pneumonia.

A third group of bacteria has a spiral or corkscrew shape. These twisted bacteria are called spirilla, and they include the bacteria that cause syphilis and some tick-borne diseases. The shape of bacteria often relates to how they move and where they can live in the human body.

What makes bacteria particularly challenging for our bodies to fight is their incredible ability to multiply. Under ideal conditions, many bacteria can double their numbers every 20 to 30 minutes. This means that one bacterium can become two, then four, then eight, and so on. In just a few hours, a small number of bacteria can grow into millions.

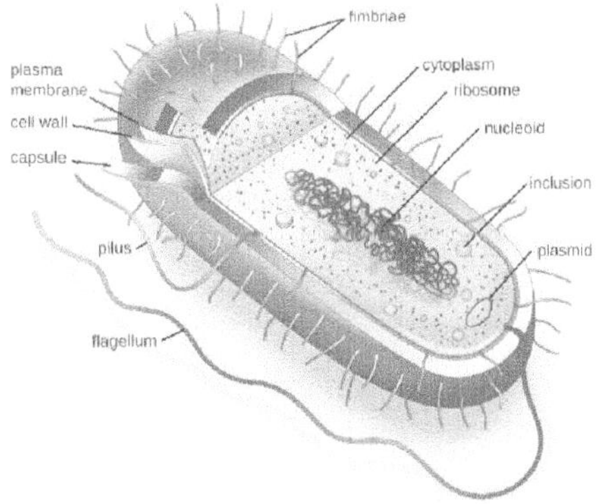

Pic 22: https://bio.libretexts.org/

This rapid multiplication explains why bacterial infections can sometimes seem to appear suddenly or get worse quickly. It also explains why early treatment of bacterial infections is often more effective than waiting until the infection has had time to establish itself.

Where They Live - Some Helpful, Some Harmful

Bacteria live virtually everywhere on Earth, from the deepest ocean trenches to the highest mountain peaks, and from frozen Antarctica to boiling hot springs. This amazing adaptability means that bacteria have also learned to live in and on the human body.

Most of the bacteria that live with us are either helpful or harmless. Your skin is home to billions of bacteria that actually protect you by taking up space and resources that harmful bacteria might otherwise use. These protective bacteria are like friendly neighbours who keep troublemakers from moving into the neighbourhood.

Inside your digestive system, helpful bacteria play crucial roles in keeping you healthy. They help break down food that your body can't digest on its own, they make certain vitamins that your body needs, and they help train your immune system to recognize the difference between friend and foe.

The bacteria in your intestines are so important that scientists sometimes call them your "second brain" because they can influence your mood, your immune system, and even your cravings for certain foods. When these good bacteria are healthy and numerous, they make it much harder for harmful bacteria to establish infections in your digestive system.

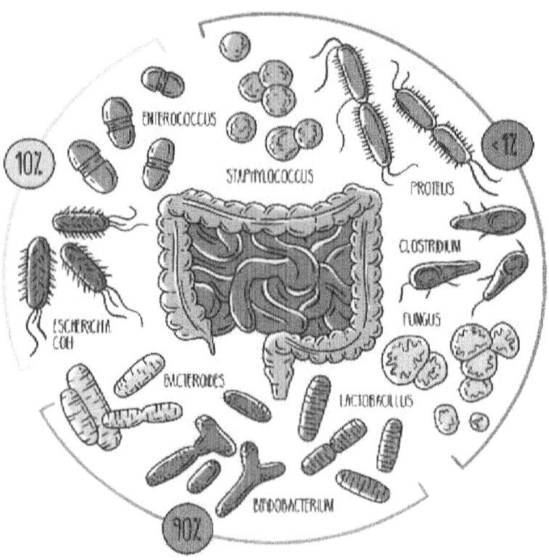

Pic 23: https://www.istockphoto.com/

However, some bacteria are definitely harmful to humans. These disease-causing bacteria, called pathogens, have developed ways to overcome our body's defences and use our bodies' resources for their own survival and reproduction.

Harmful bacteria can live in the environment around us, waiting for opportunities to enter human bodies. They might live in contaminated water, spoiled food, or in the bodies of infected animals or people. Some harmful bacteria can survive for long periods outside the human body, while others die quickly when exposed to air, heat, or cleaning agents.

How They Spread - Person to Person, Environment to Person

Understanding how bacteria spread from place to place and person to person is crucial for preventing infections. Bacteria use several different strategies to travel and find new places to live and multiply.

Direct person-to-person spread is one of the most common ways bacteria move around. This can happen through physical contact, such as shaking hands with someone who has bacteria on their skin, or through droplets that are released when someone coughs, sneezes, or even talks loudly.

When someone with a bacterial respiratory infection coughs, they release thousands of tiny droplets into the air. These droplets can contain live bacteria that can enter another person's body if they breathe them in or if the droplets land on their eyes, nose, or mouth.

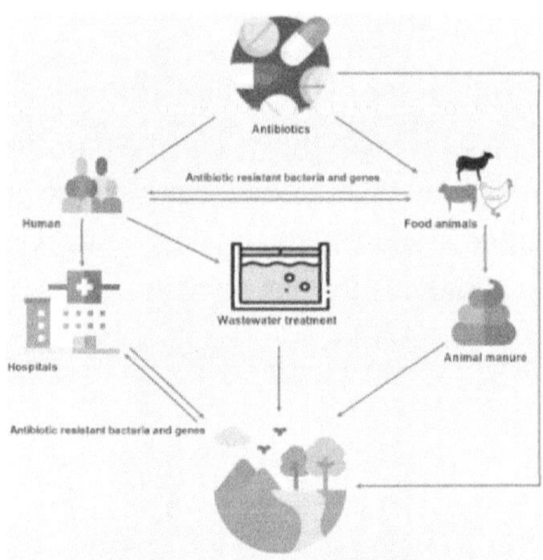

Pic 24: https://www.sciencedirect.com/

Bacteria can also spread through contaminated surfaces. If someone with bacteria on their hands touches a doorknob, phone, or eating utensil, the bacteria can survive on these surfaces for hours or even days, depending on the type of bacteria and the conditions. The next person who touches the contaminated surface can pick up the bacteria on their hands.

Food and water are major pathways for bacterial spread, especially in communities where sanitation is limited. Bacteria can contaminate food during growing, harvesting, processing, storing, or preparing. Water can become contaminated with bacteria from human or animal waste, especially when sewage systems are inadequate or when water sources are not properly protected.

Environmental spread occurs when bacteria live in soil, water, or other parts of the natural environment and then find their way into human bodies. Some bacteria can enter through broken skin when people walk barefoot on contaminated soil or swim in contaminated water.

In crowded living conditions, all of these transmission routes become more likely and more dangerous. When many people share small spaces, bacteria have more opportunities to jump from person to person. Limited access to clean water makes it harder to wash hands frequently and properly. Shared cooking and eating facilities can allow contaminated food to affect many people at once.

How Bacteria Make You Sick

Invasion and Multiplication - How They Take Over

When harmful bacteria successfully enter your body, they face the challenge of finding a place where they can survive and reproduce while avoiding your immune system's attacks. Different types of bacteria have developed different strategies for this invasion process.

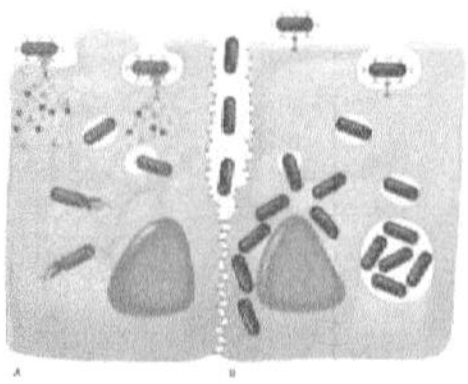

Pic 25: https://basicmedicalkey.com/

Bacterial invasion methods:

A. *The bacterial cell has an injection secretion system that is injecting multiple proteins into the host cell. Some of these cause cytoskeletal reorganization, which engulfs the bacteria. In the cytosol, the bacteria lyse the vacuolar membrane, escape, and move about.*

B. *A bacterial surface protein binds to the cell surface and induces its own endocytosis. In the cell, some escape (as in A), and others multiply in the phagosome. Another bacterium is seen invading between cells A and B by disrupting intercellular attachment molecules.*

Some bacteria are specialists that target specific parts of the body. For example, the bacteria that cause urinary tract infections are particularly good at attaching to the cells that line the urinary system. They have special structures on their surface that work like tiny grappling hooks, allowing them to grab onto these cells and resist being washed away by urine flow.

Other bacteria are more general opportunists that can cause infections in various parts of the body, depending on where they happen to land and what opportunities they find. These bacteria might cause a skin infection if they enter through a cut, a lung infection if they are breathed in, or a digestive infection if they are swallowed.

Once bacteria find a suitable place in your body, they begin the process of multiplication. They use nutrients from your body to fuel their growth and reproduction. As they multiply, they compete with your body's cells for resources like oxygen, nutrients, and space.

The speed at which bacteria multiply can quickly turn a small, manageable problem into a serious infection. This is why bacterial infections often have a characteristic pattern of getting progressively worse over hours or days, rather than staying at the same level of severity.

As bacterial populations grow, they often organize themselves into communities called biofilms. These biofilms are like bacterial cities, where the bacteria work together and protect each other from your immune system and from antibiotics. Biofilms make infections much harder to treat and explain why some bacterial infections become chronic or keep coming back.

Toxins and Damage - Why Bacterial Infections Can Be Serious

Many bacteria cause illness not just by taking up space and using resources, but also by producing toxic substances called toxins. These toxins are like bacterial weapons that can damage your body's cells and interfere with normal body functions.

Some bacteria produce toxins that directly kill cells in the area where the bacteria are growing. This cell death creates the tissue damage that we see in serious bacterial infections. For example, the bacteria that cause flesh-eating disease produce toxins that rapidly destroy skin and muscle tissue.

Other bacterial toxins interfere with specific body functions. Some toxins block nerve signals, causing paralysis. Others interfere with the digestive system, causing severe diarrhea and dehydration. Still others affect the cardiovascular system, causing dangerous drops in blood pressure.

Certain bacteria produce toxins that trigger massive inflammatory responses throughout the body. This overwhelming inflammation, called sepsis, can be life-threatening because it affects multiple organ systems at once. Sepsis is one of the reasons why bacterial infections can sometimes become medical emergencies that require immediate treatment.

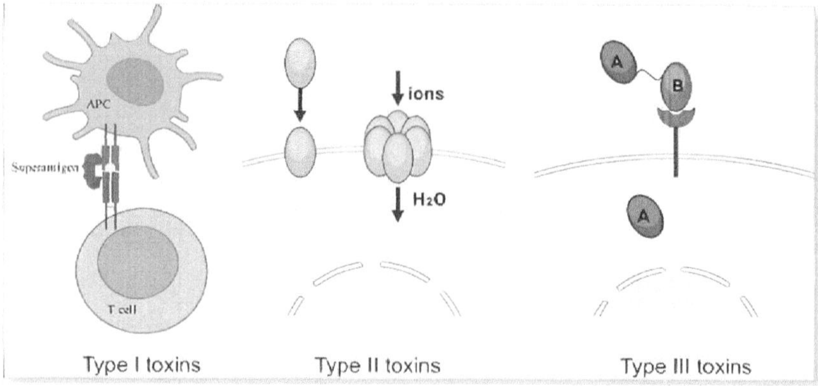

Pic 26: https://www.medsci.org/v22p2010.htm

Type I Toxins (Superantigens)

These toxins don't go inside cells but cause trouble outside. Normally, our immune system works in a very careful way: only a few T cells get activated to fight when they see a specific germ. Superantigens mess this up. They stick to both the helper T cells and the immune system's "display boards" (MHC II molecules) in a random way. This activates way too many T cells at once. As a result, huge amounts of immune chemicals, called cytokines, are released into the blood. When this happens, the body can get a high fever, nausea, vomiting, diarrhea, or even go into shock. A classic example is the toxin that causes toxic shock syndrome, made by Staphylococcus aureus.

Type II Toxins (Membrane-Damaging Toxins)

These toxins attack the cell membrane, which is like the protective wall around a cell. Some of them punch tiny holes in the membrane. Because of this, water and other things rush into the cell, causing it to swell up and eventually burst. For example, Staphylococcus aureus produces a toxin that makes holes in red blood cells. Other toxins act like chemical scissors and cut parts of the cell membrane's building blocks (phospholipids). This weakens the wall until the cell breaks apart.

Type III Toxins (A-B Toxins)

These toxins are like sneaky spies. They get inside the cell and then cause damage. They usually have two parts: part B is like the "key" that helps the toxin attach to the cell and get in, while part A is the "worker" that causes the real damage once inside. For example, the diphtheria toxin uses its B part to enter cells, and once inside, the A part shuts down protein-making machines. Without proteins, the cell can't survive

The toxins produced by bacteria can continue to cause damage even after the bacteria themselves have been killed by antibiotics or by the immune system. This is why people sometimes feel worse before they feel better during treatment for bacterial infections.

Some bacterial toxins are so potent that even very small amounts can cause serious illness. This explains why certain foodborne bacterial infections can make people severely ill even when the amount of bacteria consumed was relatively small.

Common Bacterial Infections

Pneumonia - When Bacteria Attack the Lungs

Pneumonia is one of the most serious and common bacterial infections, especially in communities where people live in crowded conditions or have limited access to healthcare. Understanding pneumonia helps explain how bacterial infections can quickly become life-threatening.

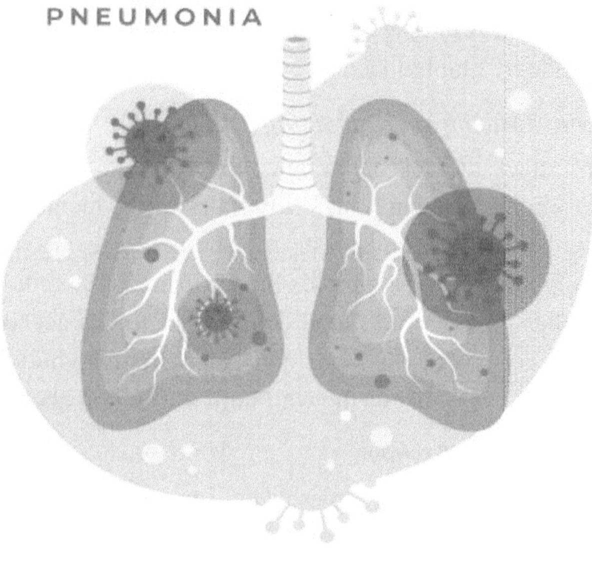

Pic 27: https://www.omegahospitals.com/

Pneumonia occurs when bacteria successfully invade the tiny air sacs in the lungs called alveoli. Normally, these air sacs are filled with air and are where oxygen enters the bloodstream and carbon dioxide is removed. When bacteria infect these air sacs, they become filled with fluid and pus instead of air.

The most common bacterial cause of pneumonia is Streptococcus pneumoniae, also called pneumococcus. This bacterium is particularly good at causing lung infections because it has a thick, slippery coating that helps it avoid being destroyed by the immune system's initial defenses.

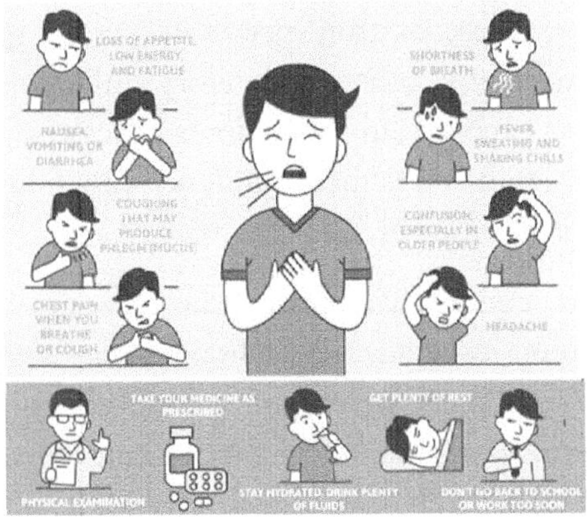

Pic 28: https://www.fasttrackurgentcare.com/

People with bacterial pneumonia typically develop symptoms over a period of hours to days. They may start with what feels like a cold or flu, but then develop a high fever, chills, and a cough that produces thick, colored sputum. The infected person may also experience chest pain, especially when breathing deeply or coughing.

As pneumonia progresses, the person may have difficulty breathing because the infected air sacs can't effectively exchange oxygen and carbon dioxide. In severe cases, the lack of oxygen can affect other organs, including the heart and brain.

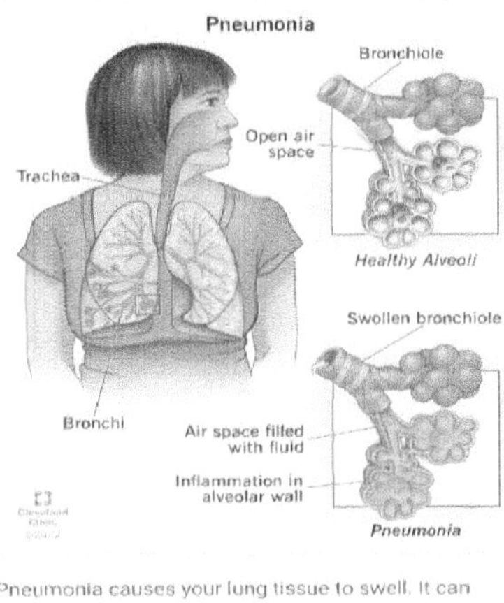

Pic 29: https://edurev.in/t/381326/NCERT-Summary- Human-Health-and-Diseases

Bacterial pneumonia spreads from person to person through respiratory droplets, just like many other respiratory infections. However, not everyone who is exposed to pneumonia bacteria will develop the infection. People with weakened immune systems, underlying lung conditions, or poor nutrition are at higher risk.

In crowded living conditions, pneumonia can spread rapidly through families or communities. Poor ventilation increases the risk because it allows respiratory droplets to remain in the air longer. Exposure to smoke from cooking fires or other sources can damage the lungs and make pneumonia more likely.

Urinary Tract Infections (UTIs) - Bacteria in the Urinary System

Urinary tract infections are among the most common bacterial infections, affecting millions of people worldwide. These infections occur when bacteria that normally live harmlessly in other parts of the body find their way into the urinary system and begin multiplying.

The urinary system includes the kidneys, which filter waste from the blood; the ureters, which carry urine from the kidneys to the bladder; the bladder, which stores urine; and the urethra, which carries urine out of the body. Bacteria can cause infections in any part of this system, but infections of the bladder and urethra are most common.

Most urinary tract infections are caused by bacteria called Escherichia coli, or E. coli for short. These bacteria normally live harmlessly in the intestines, where they actually help with digestion. However, when E. coli bacteria travel from the intestinal area to the urinary tract, they can cause infection.

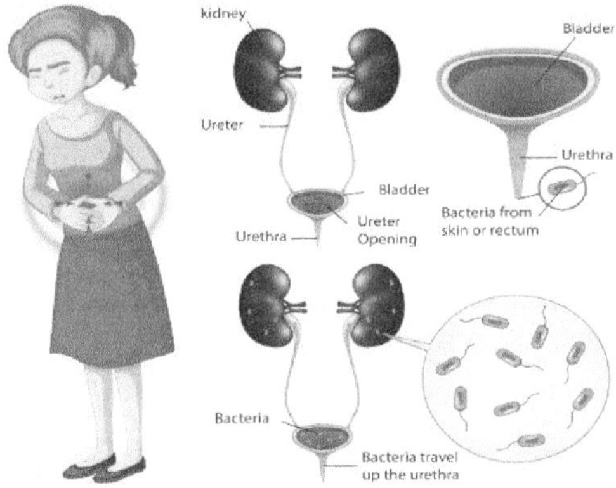

Pic 30: https://drmanasabadveli.com/

Women are much more likely to develop urinary tract infections than men because of anatomy. The female urethra is shorter than the male urethra, which means bacteria don't have to travel as far to reach the bladder. The opening of the female urethra is also closer to the anal area, where intestinal bacteria normally live.

Symptoms of urinary tract infections include a burning sensation during urination, frequent urges to urinate even when the bladder is not full, cloudy or strong-smelling urine, and pelvic pain in women. Some people may also develop fever and back pain, especially if the infection spreads to the kidneys.

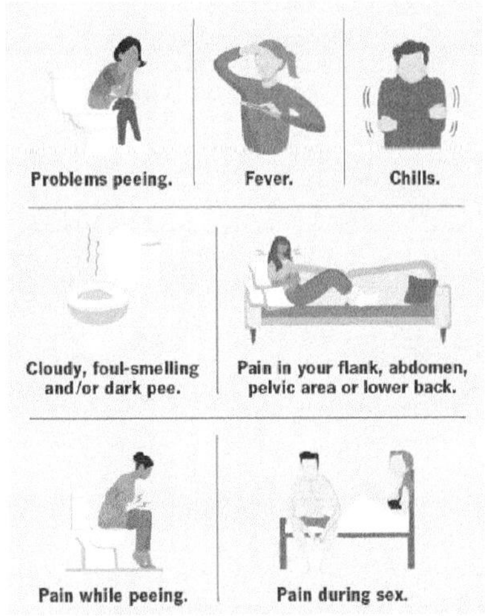

Pic 31: https://my.clevelandclinic.org/

In communities with limited access to clean water and adequate toilet facilities, urinary tract infections can be more common and more serious. Poor hygiene practices can increase the chance that bacteria will spread from the intestinal area to the urinary tract. Holding urine for long periods because of inadequate toilet facilities can also increase infection risk.

Wound Infections - When Cuts Get Infected

Any break in the skin, from a tiny scratch to a major cut, creates an opportunity for bacteria to enter the body. While most small wounds heal without problems, understanding how wound infections develop helps explain when to be concerned and when to seek help.

Normal, healthy skin is an excellent barrier against bacterial invasion. The skin's surface is slightly acidic and dry, conditions that many harmful bacteria cannot tolerate. The skin also constantly sheds its outer layer, taking away any bacteria that might be trying to establish themselves.

When the skin is broken, even by a small cut or scrape, bacteria can enter the body through the opening. The type and severity of wound infection that develops depends on several factors: the type and number of bacteria that enter the wound, the depth and size of the wound, and the person's general health and immune system strength.

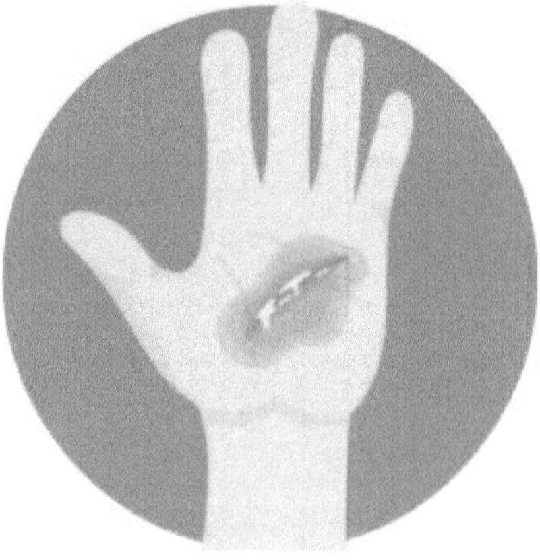

Pic 32: https://www.shutterstock.com/

The most common bacteria that cause wound infections are Staphylococcus aureus (staph) and Streptococcus pyogenes (strep). Staph bacteria normally live on the skin and in the nose of many healthy people without causing problems. However, when staph bacteria enter a wound, they can cause infections ranging from minor skin irritation to serious, life-threatening conditions.

Signs of wound infection include increasing redness around the wound, warmth, swelling, pain that gets worse instead of better, and the development of pus. Red streaks extending away from the wound are a particularly concerning sign that suggests the infection may be spreading through the lymphatic system.

In crowded living conditions, wound infections can be more common and more serious for several reasons. Limited access to clean water makes it difficult to properly clean wounds when they occur. Crowded conditions mean that wounds are more likely to come into contact with bacteria from other people or from contaminated surfaces.

Poor nutrition can slow wound healing and make infections more likely. When the body lacks the protein, vitamins, and minerals needed for tissue repair, even small wounds may heal slowly and become infected.

Foodborne Bacterial Infections - Contaminated Food and Water

Foodborne bacterial infections, often called food poisoning, occur when people consume food or water that contains harmful bacteria. These infections can range from mild stomach upset to severe, life-threatening illness, depending on the type and amount of bacteria consumed.

Several different types of bacteria can cause foodborne illness. Salmonella bacteria are among the most common causes, often found in contaminated eggs, poultry, and dairy products. Campylobacter bacteria frequently contaminate poultry and can cause severe diarrhea. E. coli bacteria, particularly certain strains, can cause serious illness when they contaminate ground beef or fresh produce.

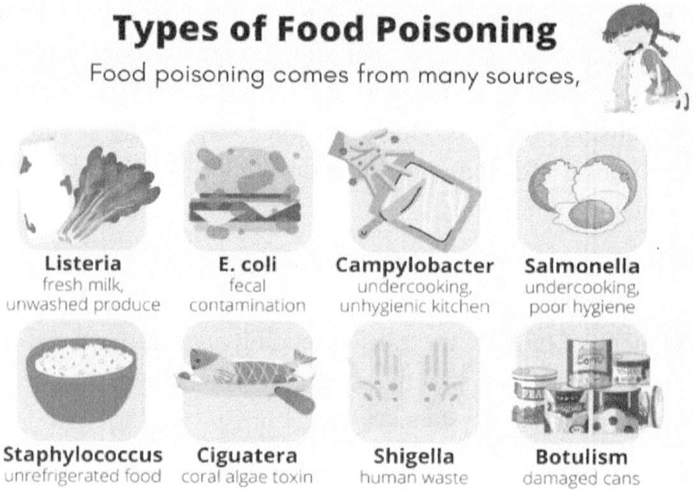
Types of Food Poisoning
Food poisoning comes from many sources,
Listeria
fresh milk,
unwashed produce
E. coli
fecal
contamination
Campylobacter
undercooking,
unhygienic kitchen
Salmonella
undercooking,
poor hygiene
Staphylococcus
unrefrigerated food
Ciguatera
coral algae toxin
Shigella
human waste
Botulism
damaged cans

Pic 33: https://sciencenotes.org/

Food can become contaminated with bacteria at many points from farm to table. Animals used for food may carry bacteria in their intestines without appearing sick. During slaughter and processing, bacteria from the intestines can contaminate meat. Fresh produce can become contaminated if it's irrigated with water that contains animal waste or if it's handled by people with contaminated hands.

In communities with limited refrigeration, food contamination becomes a greater risk because bacteria multiply rapidly at warm temperatures. Street food vendors may lack access to clean water for washing hands and utensils. Inadequate cooking facilities may not reach temperatures hot enough to kill bacteria.

Symptoms of foodborne bacterial infections typically include nausea, vomiting, diarrhea, stomach cramps, and sometimes fever. These symptoms usually develop within a few hours to a few days after eating contaminated food. Most people recover within a few days, but some bacterial foodborne infections can cause serious complications.

The key to preventing foodborne bacterial infections is breaking the chain of contamination. This includes keeping food at safe temperatures, cooking food to temperatures hot enough to kill bacteria, avoiding cross contamination between raw and cooked foods, and maintaining good hygiene during food preparation.

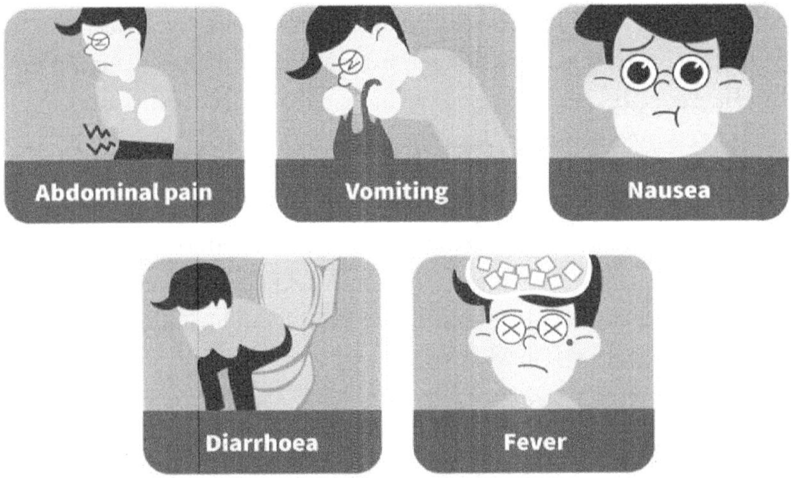

Pic 34: https://www.cfs.gov.hk/

Recognizing Bacterial Infections

Common Signs - Pus, Prolonged Fever, Localized Pain

Learning to recognize the signs of bacterial infections can help you know when to seek treatment and when home care might be sufficient. Bacterial infections often have characteristic features that distinguish them from viral infections or other health problems.

Pus formation is one of the most distinctive signs of bacterial infection. Pus is a thick, usually yellowish or greenish fluid that forms when white blood cells fight bacteria. The pus contains dead bacteria, dead white blood cells, and fluid from the surrounding tissues. While pus formation shows that your immune system is actively fighting infection, it also indicates that bacteria are present in significant numbers.

Pus can form anywhere in the body where bacterial infection occurs. It may be visible in infected wounds, or it may be coughed up from infected lungs, or it may cause cloudy urine in urinary tract infections. The presence of pus usually indicates that antibiotic treatment will be helpful.

Prolonged or recurring fever is another important sign of bacterial infection. While viral infections can also cause fever, bacterial infections often cause fever that lasts longer or that returns after seeming to go away. Bacterial fevers may also be higher than viral fevers and may be accompanied by chills and sweating.

The pattern of fever can provide clues about what type of infection is present. A fever that rises and falls in a regular pattern might suggest a different type of bacterial infection than a fever that remains constantly high. Fever that develops gradually over days might indicate a different problem than fever that appears suddenly.

Localized pain and inflammation are common features of bacterial infections. Unlike viral infections, which often cause general feelings of illness, bacterial infections frequently cause pain and inflammation in the specific area where the bacteria are growing.

For example, bacterial skin infections cause pain, redness, warmth, and swelling in the affected area. Bacterial ear infections cause ear pain that may be severe. Bacterial urinary tract infections cause pain during urination and sometimes back or pelvic pain.

Why Bacterial Infections Often Get Worse Without Treatment

Bacterial infections have a tendency to worsen over time if they are not properly treated. This progression occurs because bacteria continue to multiply and spread, overwhelming the body's natural defenses.

Unlike viral infections, which often improve on their own as the immune system learns to fight the virus, bacterial infections can continue indefinitely. The bacteria keep reproducing and consuming resources, and they may spread to new areas of the body.

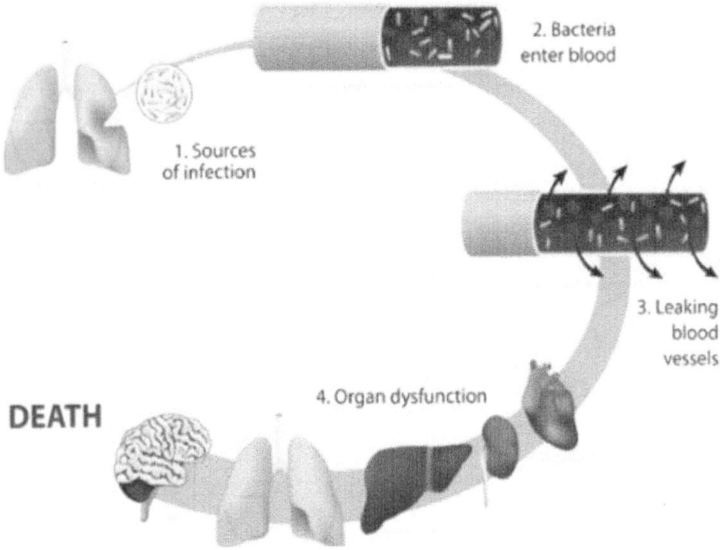

Pic 35: https://www.drkarunhematology.com/

As bacterial populations grow, they can cause increasing tissue damage. The toxins produced by bacteria can kill healthy cells and interfere with normal body functions. The immune system's response to large numbers of bacteria can cause inflammation that damages healthy tissue along with infected tissue.

Untreated bacterial infections can also spread beyond their original location. Bacteria can enter the bloodstream and travel to other parts of the body, causing new infections in multiple organs. This spreading, called bacteremia or sepsis, can be life- threatening.

The formation of biofilms makes bacterial infections increasingly difficult to treat the longer they persist. As bacteria organize into these protective communities, they become more resistant to both the immune system and to antibiotic treatments.

Early treatment of bacterial infections is usually more effective than delayed treatment. When bacterial populations are still small, antibiotics can more easily eliminate them. The immune system can also more effectively clear small numbers of bacteria than large, established populations.

Laboratory Tests - When and Why They Help

Laboratory tests can provide valuable information about bacterial infections, helping to identify the specific type of bacteria causing illness and determining which antibiotics will be most effective. However, these tests are not always necessary or available, especially in resource-limited settings.

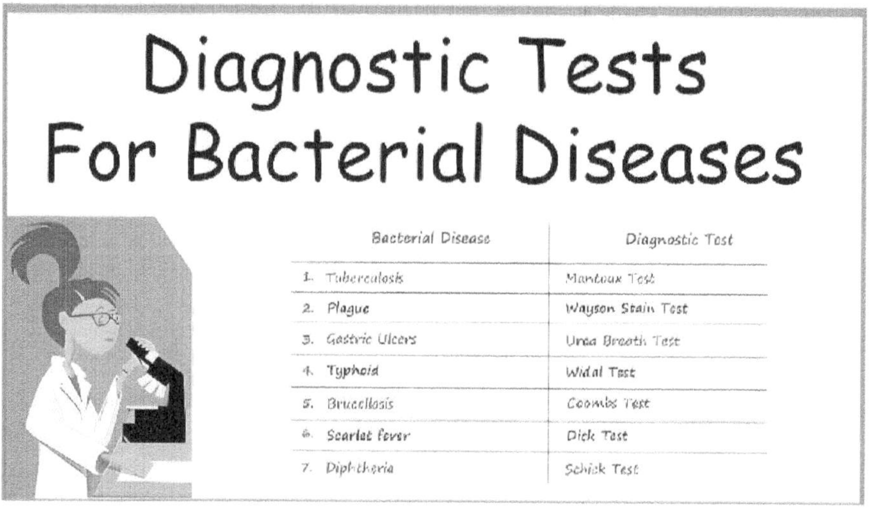

Pic 36: https://www.youtube.com/watch?v=Ft73z5etxgo

Culture tests involve taking a sample from the infected area and growing any bacteria present in a laboratory. This allows identification of the specific bacterial species and testing of which antibiotics can kill those particular bacteria. Culture tests are most useful for serious infections, infections that don't respond to initial treatment, or infections in areas where antibiotic resistance is common.

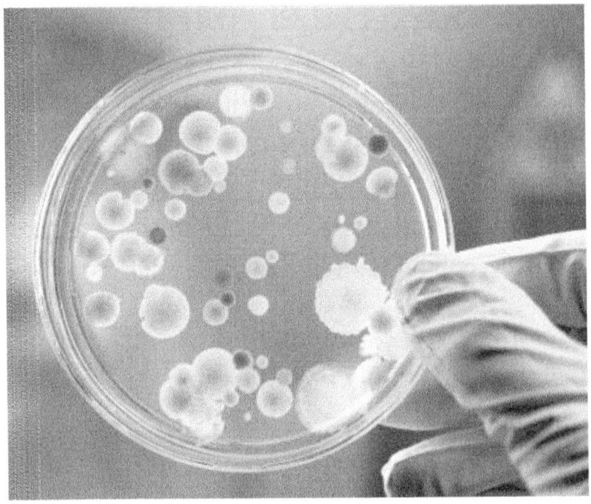

Pic 37: https://www.doghealth.com/

Blood tests can help determine how serious a bacterial infection is and whether it has spread throughout the body. A complete blood count can show whether the number of white blood cells is elevated, which often occurs during bacterial infections. Other blood tests can measure markers of inflammation or organ function.

Urine tests are commonly used to diagnose urinary tract infections. These tests can quickly identify bacteria and white blood cells in the urine, confirming the presence of infection. More detailed urine cultures can identify the specific bacteria and guide antibiotic selection.

While laboratory tests can be very helpful, they are not always necessary for diagnosing and treating common bacterial infections. Many bacterial infections can be diagnosed based on symptoms and physical examination alone. In communities with limited access to laboratory facilities, healthcare providers often need to make treatment decisions based on clinical judgment.

The cost and availability of laboratory tests must be balanced against their potential benefits. For minor infections that are likely to respond to standard treatments, tests may not be cost-effective. For serious infections or infections that don't respond to initial treatment, laboratory tests can be life-saving.

Antibiotics: The Bacterial Fighters

How Antibiotics Work - Killing or Stopping Bacteria

Antibiotics are medicines specifically designed to fight bacterial infections. They work by targeting aspects of bacterial cells that are different from human cells, allowing them to kill bacteria without severely harming the person taking them.

Different antibiotics work through different mechanisms. Some antibiotics attack the bacterial cell wall, which is a structure that bacteria have but human cells lack. These antibiotics cause the bacterial cell wall to break down, killing the bacteria. Penicillin and related antibiotics work this way.

Other antibiotics interfere with bacterial protein production. Bacteria need to make proteins to survive and reproduce, just like all living things. Some antibiotics block the machinery that bacteria use to make proteins, effectively starving the bacteria to death.

Still other antibiotics interfere with bacterial DNA replication. Since bacteria reproduce by copying their DNA and dividing into two cells, antibiotics that prevent DNA copying can stop bacterial reproduction even if they don't immediately kill existing bacteria.

Some antibiotics work by disrupting the bacterial cell membrane, which controls what goes in and out of the bacterial cell. When this membrane is damaged, essential materials leak out of the bacterial cell and harmful substances can enter, killing the bacteria.

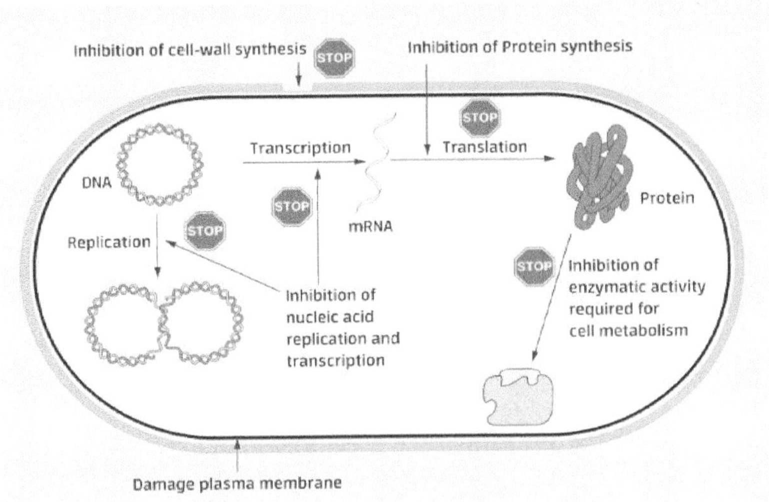

Pic 38: https://everythingaboutbiotech.tumblr.com/

The fact that antibiotics target structures or processes that are specific to bacteria is what makes them relatively safe for humans. However, this also explains why antibiotics don't work against viruses, which have very different structures and reproduction mechanisms.

Understanding how antibiotics work helps explain why it's important to take them exactly as prescribed. Taking too little antibiotic may not kill all the bacteria, allowing the strongest ones to survive and multiply. Taking antibiotics for too short a time may allow bacteria to recover and cause the infection to return.

When Antibiotics Help - Right Infections, Right Time

Antibiotics are powerful tools for treating bacterial infections, but they are only helpful when used for the right type of infection at the right time. Using antibiotics appropriately maximizes their benefits while minimizing potential harm.

Antibiotics are most effective when used early in the course of a bacterial infection, before the bacteria have had time to multiply extensively or form protective biofilms. Early treatment can often cure infections quickly and prevent complications.

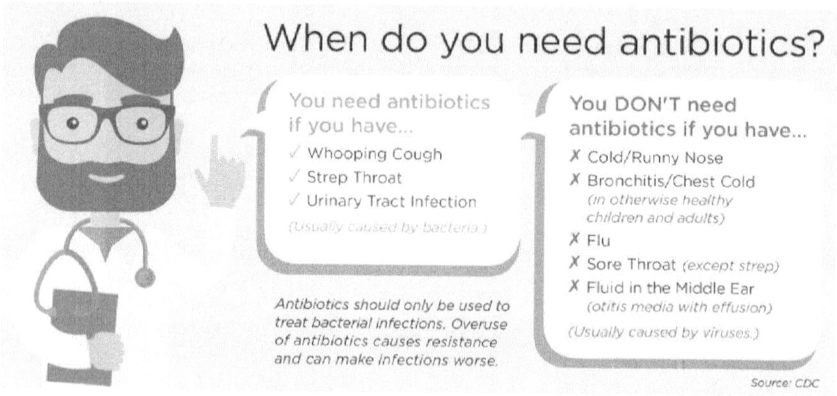

Pic 39: https://www.cedars-sinai.org/

However, not all bacterial infections require antibiotic treatment. Many minor bacterial infections, such as small skin infections, can be successfully treated with local care like cleaning and bandaging. The body's immune system can often eliminate small numbers of bacteria without assistance.

The decision about whether to use antibiotics should consider the severity of the infection, the risk of complications, and the person's overall health. Serious bacterial infections like pneumonia or bloodstream infections almost always require antibiotic treatment. Minor infections in healthy people may be successfully treated without antibiotics.

The specific type of antibiotic used should be chosen based on the type of bacteria causing the infection and the location of the infection in the body. Some antibiotics work well against certain types of bacteria but not others. Some antibiotics reach high concentrations in certain parts of the body but not in others.

When laboratory testing is available, culture and sensitivity testing can help guide antibiotic selection by identifying the specific bacteria and determining which antibiotics will be most effective. When testing is not available, healthcare providers choose antibiotics based on their knowledge of which bacteria commonly cause particular types of infections.

When Antibiotics Don't Work - Viral Infections, Wrong Type

One of the most important concepts in medicine is understanding when antibiotics will not be helpful. Misusing antibiotics not only wastes resources but can also cause harm and contribute to the development of antibiotic-resistant bacteria.

Bacterial cells have cell walls, which are rigid structures that protect the bacteria and give them their shape. Many antibiotics work by preventing bacteria from building or maintaining these cell walls. Without functional cell walls, bacteria cannot survive.

However, viruses don't have cell walls at all, so antibiotics that target cell walls have no effect on them.

Bacteria have their own protein-making machinery, including ribosomes that are different from human ribosomes. Some antibiotics specifically target bacterial ribosomes, preventing bacteria from making the proteins they need to survive. Viruses don't have their own ribosomes - they hijack human ribosomes to make viral proteins, so antibiotics that target bacterial ribosomes don't affect viral reproduction.

Many antibiotics interfere with bacterial DNA replication or repair. Bacteria have circular DNA molecules that are packaged and replicated differently than human DNA. Viruses have various types of genetic material, including DNA and RNA, but they use the host cell's machinery for replication, making them immune to antibiotics that target bacterial DNA processes.

Some antibiotics work by interfering with bacterial metabolism - the chemical processes that bacteria use to generate energy and build cellular components.

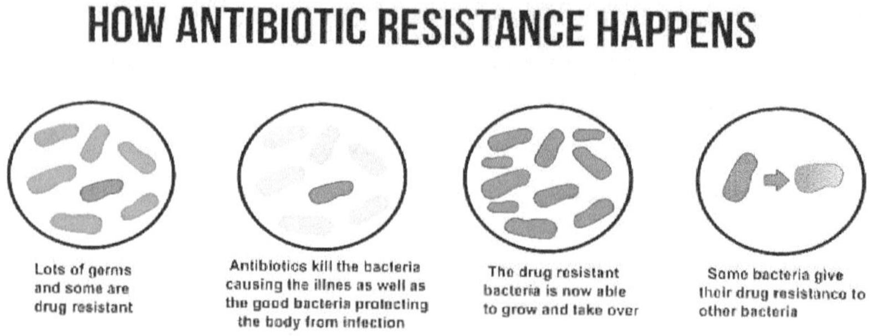

Pic 40: https://www.shutterstock.com/

Unnecessary antibiotic use also contributes to the broader problem of antibiotic resistance in communities. When antibiotics are used frequently, bacteria are under constant pressure to develop resistance. Resistant bacteria can then spread from person to person, making infections harder to treat for everyone.

Community Focus: Preventing Antibiotic Resistance

Antibiotic resistance is a growing global health threat that particularly affects communities with limited healthcare resources. Understanding how resistance develops and spreads helps explain why community-wide action is needed to preserve the effectiveness of these life-saving medicines.

Complete the Full Course

Taking the complete course of antibiotics as prescribed is one of the most important steps individuals can take to prevent resistance. When people stop taking antibiotics as soon as they feel better, some bacteria may still be alive in their bodies. These surviving bacteria are often the strongest ones that were most resistant to the antibiotic.

If these resistant bacteria continue to multiply, they can cause the infection to return, but now the same antibiotic may not work as well. These resistant bacteria can also spread to other people, who may then develop infections that are harder to treat.

Completing the full course of antibiotics, even after symptoms improve, helps ensure that all bacteria are eliminated. This reduces the chance that resistant bacteria will survive and multiply.

Don't Share Antibiotics

Sharing antibiotics between family members or friends is dangerous for several reasons. Different people may need different types or amounts of antibiotics, even for infections that seem similar. What works for one person may not work for another.

Shared antibiotics may not provide enough medicine to completely cure an infection, leading to the survival of resistant bacteria. The person sharing the antibiotic may also not have enough medicine to complete their own treatment properly.

Don't Pressure Doctors for Antibiotics

Understanding when antibiotics are and are not helpful allows patients to work with healthcare providers to make appropriate treatment decisions. Pressuring healthcare providers to prescribe antibiotics for viral infections or minor bacterial infections that don't require treatment contributes to inappropriate antibiotic use.

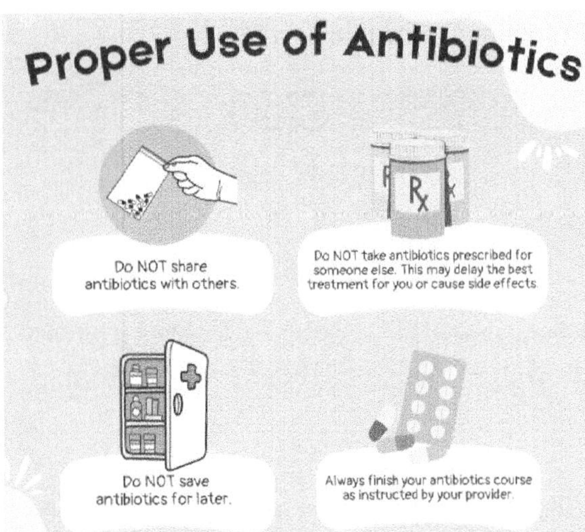

Pic 41: https://www.instagram.com/p/Cz30LLUPkv5/?img_inde x=2

Building trust with healthcare providers and understanding their reasoning for treatment recommendations helps ensure that antibiotics are used only when they will be beneficial.

Dangers of Fake/Expired Antibiotics in Slums

In many communities with limited access to healthcare, counterfeit or expired antibiotics may be sold at lower prices than genuine medicines. These fake medicines pose serious dangers to both individual health and community antibiotic resistance.

Counterfeit antibiotics may contain no active ingredient at all, wrong ingredients, or the correct ingredients in wrong amounts. People who take fake antibiotics may think they are being treated while their infections continue to worsen.

Expired antibiotics may have reduced effectiveness, providing enough antibiotic pressure to select for resistant bacteria but not enough to cure infections. This creates ideal conditions for the development and spread of antibiotic resistance.

Learning to identify reliable sources of genuine antibiotics and understanding the importance of proper storage helps protect both individual and community health.

Chapter - 6
Viral Infections - The Hijackers

"Viruses: the tiniest troublemakers"

What Makes Viruses Different

Size Comparison - Much Smaller Than Bacteria

Viruses represent a completely different category of infectious agent from bacteria, and understanding these differences is crucial for knowing how to prevent and treat viral infections. The most obvious difference is size - viruses are incredibly tiny, even compared to bacteria.

If bacteria are small enough that thousands could fit across a human hair, viruses are so small that hundreds of them could fit inside a single bacterium. To put this in perspective, if a virus were the size of a marble, a bacterium would be the size of a basketball, and a human cell would be the size of a large building.

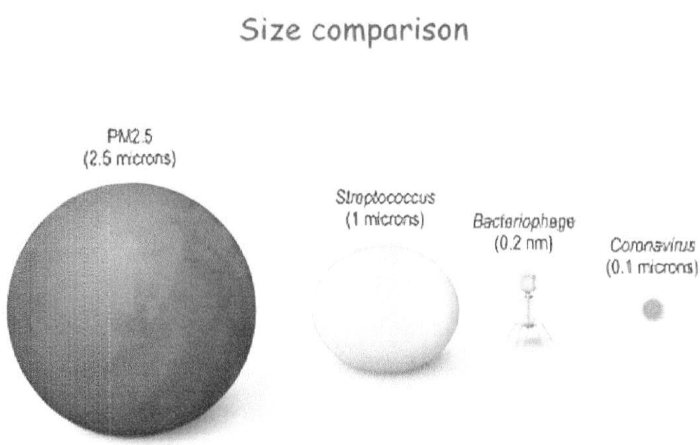

Pic 42: https://www.shutterstock.com/

This extreme small size means that viruses can penetrate barriers that might stop bacteria. They can pass through filters that block bacteria, and they can fit into spaces in the body where bacteria cannot go. Their tiny size also makes them extremely difficult to see, even with powerful microscopes.

The small size of viruses also affects how they spread. Because they are so light, viral particles can remain suspended in air for longer periods than bacteria. They can travel further when people cough or sneeze, and they can be carried by air currents throughout buildings.

Despite their tiny size, viruses can cause diseases that are just as serious as bacterial infections, and sometimes more serious. The COVID-19 pandemic demonstrated how a virus invisible to the naked eye could affect the entire world.

How Viruses Work - Hijacking Your Cells to Multiply

Perhaps the most important difference between viruses and bacteria is how they reproduce. While bacteria are complete, independent cells that can reproduce on their own, viruses are essentially genetic material wrapped in a protein coat. They cannot reproduce without taking over the machinery of living cells.

Think of viruses as extremely sophisticated pirates. They cannot sail their own ships or gather their own food, but they are experts at taking over other ships and forcing the crew to work for them.

Once a virus hijacks a cell, it forces that cell to stop doing its normal job and instead focus on making copies of the virus.

The process begins when a virus attaches to the outside of a cell. Different viruses are designed to attach to different types of cells. Cold viruses typically attach to cells in the nose and throat, while stomach viruses attach to cells in the digestive system.

Once attached, the virus injects its genetic material into the cell. This genetic material contains instructions for making new viruses. The virus essentially reprograms the cell, forcing it to use its energy and resources to manufacture viral components instead of maintaining itself.

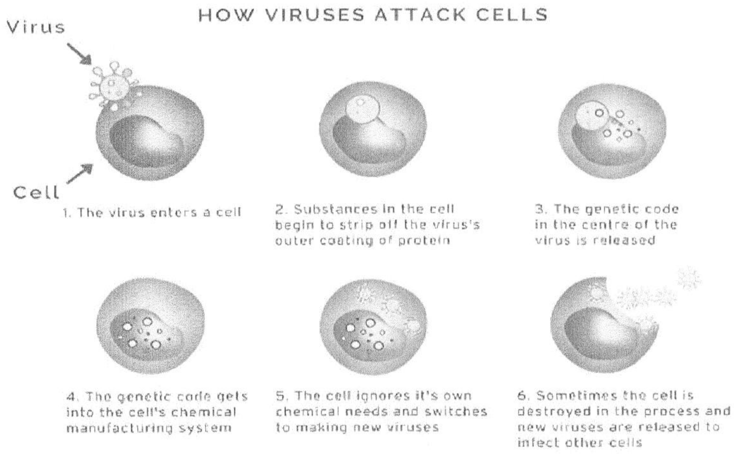

Pic 43: https://www.facebook.com/UnderstandingAnimalResearch

The hijacked cell becomes a virus factory, producing hundreds or thousands of new viral particles. Eventually, the cell becomes so full of new viruses that it bursts open, releasing the new viruses to infect other cells. Alternatively, some viruses bud off from the cell surface, gradually weakening the cell while producing new viruses.

This hijacking process explains why viral infections often make people feel so sick. As more and more cells are hijacked and destroyed, normal body functions become impaired. The immune system's response to viral infection can also cause many of the symptoms we associate with being sick.

Why Viruses Are Harder to Treat - Living Inside Your Cells

The fact that viruses live and reproduce inside human cells makes them much more difficult to treat than bacterial infections. Any medicine that kills viruses must be able to get inside human cells, and it must be able to distinguish between viral components and human cellular components.

This is a much more challenging task than killing bacteria, which live outside human cells and have many structures that are completely different from human cells. Most antiviral medicines work by interfering with specific steps in the viral reproduction process, but these medicines are often less effective than antibiotics and may have more side effects.

Because viruses use the host cell's machinery to reproduce, stopping viral reproduction often requires interfering with normal cellular processes. This can damage human cells along with viruses, leading to side effects from antiviral medications.

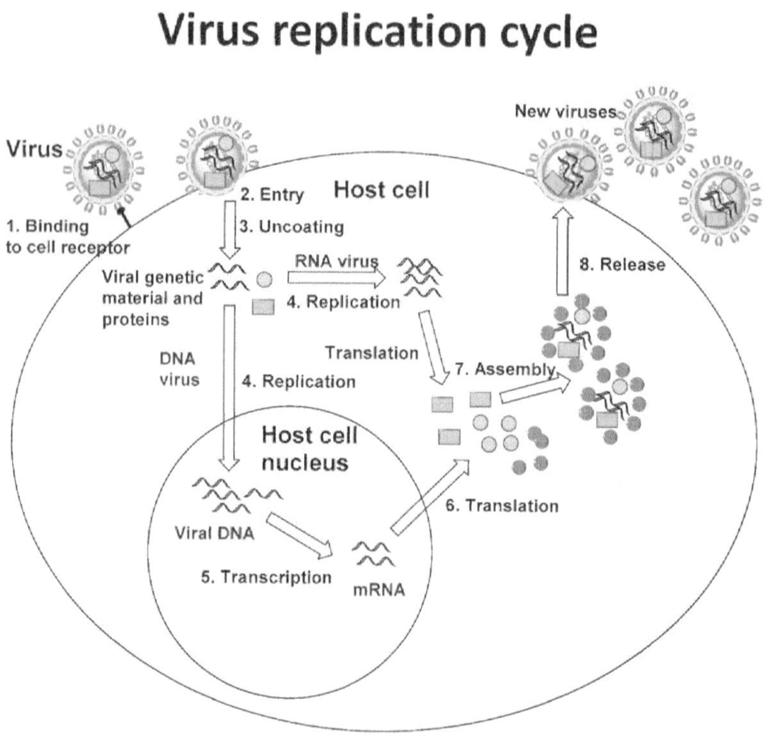

Pic 44: https://www.mdpi.com/1999-4915/13/4/667

Another challenge in treating viral infections is that viruses can change rapidly. Many viruses have high mutation rates, meaning they frequently develop genetic changes that can make them resistant to antiviral medicines. The influenza virus, for example, changes so rapidly that new vaccines must be developed each year.

Some viruses can also remain dormant inside cells for long periods, hidden from both the immune system and antiviral medicines. These latent viruses can reactivate later, causing new symptoms even years after the initial infection.

Common Viral Infections in Our Communities Respiratory Viruses

Common Cold - The Everyday Annoyance

The common cold is probably the most frequent viral infection experienced by humans worldwide. Despite its name suggesting a single disease, the common cold is actually caused by many different viruses, with **rhinoviruses** being the most common culprits.

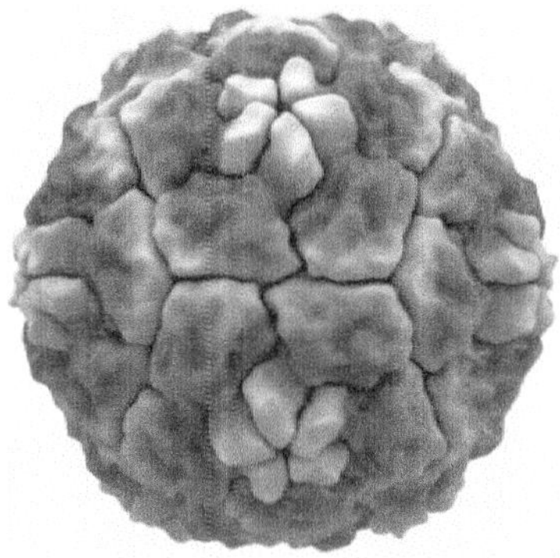

Pic 45: https://en.wikipedia.org/wiki/Rhinovirus

Cold viruses primarily infect the cells lining the nose and throat. When these cells are hijacked by viruses, they become inflamed and produce excess mucus as part of the immune response. This inflammation and mucus production cause the familiar symptoms of stuffy nose, runny nose, sneezing, and sore throat.

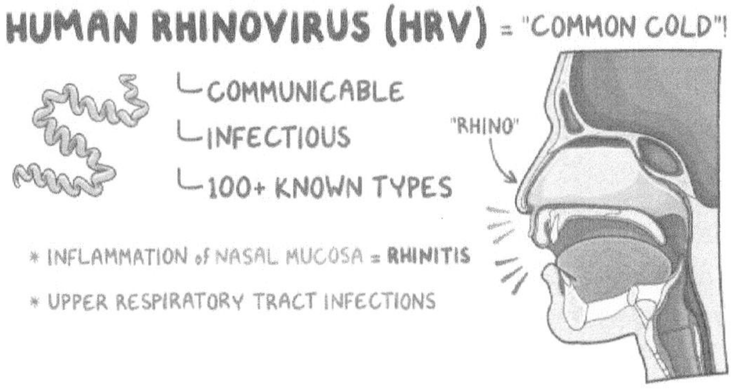

Pic 46: https://www.osmosis.org/learn/Rhinovirus

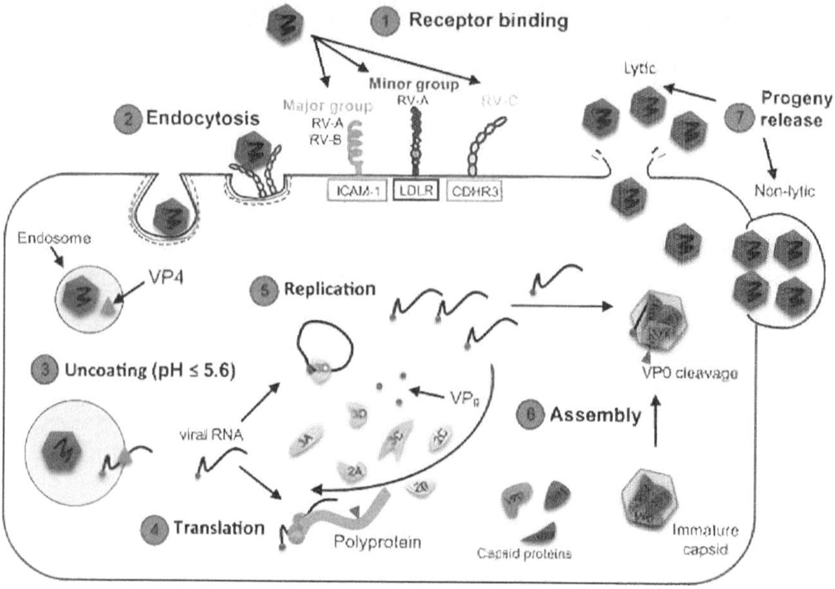

Pic 47: https://www.sciencedirect.com/topics/agricultural-and-biological-sciences/rhinovirus-c

Stage-by-Stage Rhinovirus Infection

Stage 1 (Receptor Binding): *The rhinovirus floats through the air or on your hands until it encounters cells lining your nose and throat, where it attaches to specific receptor proteins on the cell surface like a key fitting into a lock.*

Stage 2 (Endocytosis): *The cell membrane wraps around the virus and pulls it inside the cell through a process called endocytosis, essentially swallowing the virus whole.*

Stage 3 (Uncoating): *Once inside the cell, the acidic environment causes the virus to shed its protective protein coat and release its RNA genetic material into the cell's interior.*

Stage 4 (Replication): *The viral RNA hijacks the cell's machinery and forces it to make thousands of copies of the virus's genetic material instead of doing its normal cellular work.*

Stage 5 (Translation): *The cell's ribosomes read the viral RNA instructions and manufacture all the proteins needed to build new virus particles.*

Stage 6 (Assembly): *The newly made viral proteins and RNA copies come together like pieces of a puzzle to form complete, infectious rhinovirus particles inside the cell.*

Lytic vs Non-Lytic Release

Lytic Release: *The cell becomes so packed with new viruses that it bursts open like an overstuffed balloon, immediately releasing hundreds of new rhinoviruses that can infect nearby cells. This kills the host cell instantly.*

Non-Lytic Release: *New viruses bud off from the cell membrane gradually, wrapping themselves in pieces of the cell's outer layer as they leave, which allows the infected cell to stay alive longer and continue producing more viruses over time.*

Rhinovirus typically uses the lytic pathway, which is why your nose and throat cells get damaged during a cold, leading to inflammation and those uncomfortable cold symptoms.

Most adults experience two to three colds per year, while children may have six to eight colds annually. Children get more colds because their immune systems haven't yet encountered many of the viruses that cause colds, and because they often have close contact with other children who may be infected.

Cold symptoms typically develop gradually over one to three days after exposure to the virus. The illness usually peaks around day three or four and then gradually improves over the following week. Unlike more serious viral infections, colds rarely cause high fever in adults, though children may develop low-grade fevers.

In crowded living conditions, cold viruses spread very easily from person to person. When someone with a cold coughs, sneezes, or even talks, they release thousands of tiny droplets containing viruses into the air. Other people can become infected by breathing these droplets or by touching surfaces where the droplets have landed and then touching their nose, mouth, or eyes.

While colds are generally mild and resolve on their own, they can sometimes lead to secondary bacterial infections, particularly in people with underlying health conditions. Sinus infections and ear infections are common bacterial complications of viral colds.

Influenza (Flu) - The Seasonal Threat

Influenza, commonly called the flu, is a more serious viral infection than the common cold. Flu viruses infect the respiratory system but typically cause more severe symptoms and can lead to serious complications, especially in vulnerable populations.

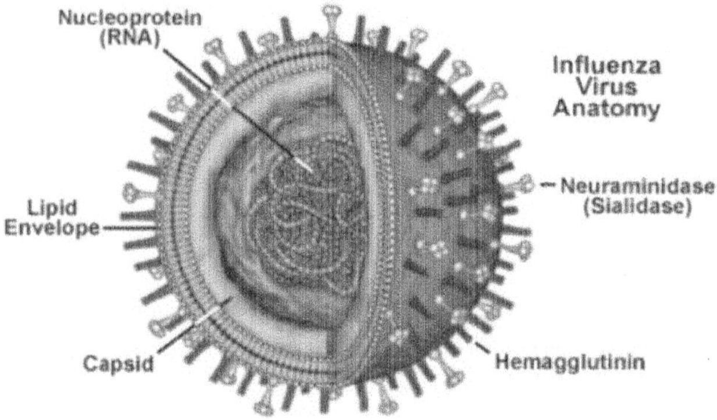

Pic 48: https://micro.magnet.fsu.edu/cells/viruses/influenzavirus.html

There are three main types of influenza viruses that affect humans: influenza A, influenza B, and influenza C. Influenza A viruses are generally the most serious and are responsible for seasonal flu epidemics and pandemic outbreaks. These viruses are constantly changing, which is why people can get the flu multiple times and why annual flu vaccines are necessary.

Flu symptoms typically come on suddenly, unlike cold symptoms which develop gradually. People with flu often experience high fever, severe headache, muscle aches throughout the body, extreme fatigue, and dry cough. The fever and body aches can be quite severe, often forcing people to stay in bed for several days.

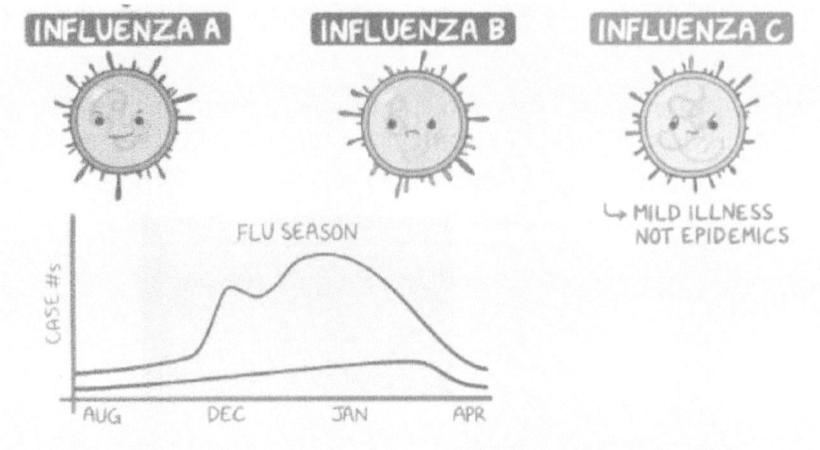

Pic 49: https://www.osmosis.org/learn/Influenza_virus

The flu season typically occurs during cooler months when people spend more time indoors in close contact with others. In crowded living conditions, flu can spread rapidly through families and communities. Poor ventilation increases the risk of transmission because viral particles can remain suspended in the air for extended periods.

Influenza can cause serious complications, particularly in young children, adults over 65, pregnant women, and people with underlying health conditions like asthma, diabetes, or heart disease. These complications can include pneumonia, which can be life-threatening.

Prevention of influenza relies primarily on vaccination when available, and on the same hygiene measures used to prevent other respiratory viruses. Because flu viruses change frequently, previous infection or vaccination may not provide complete protection against new flu strains.

COVID-19 - The Pandemic Virus

The COVID-19 pandemic, caused by the SARS-CoV-2 virus, has demonstrated how a new viral infection can rapidly spread around the world and significantly impact communities, especially those with limited healthcare resources.

COVID-19 symptoms can range from very mild to severe and life-threatening. Many people with COVID-19 experience fever, cough, shortness of breath, fatigue, muscle aches, loss of taste or smell, sore throat, and headache. Some people, particularly children, may have no symptoms at all but can still spread the virus to others.

What makes COVID-19 particularly challenging is that people can spread the virus to others even before they develop symptoms, or even if they never develop symptoms. This silent transmission has made it difficult to control the spread of the virus through communities.

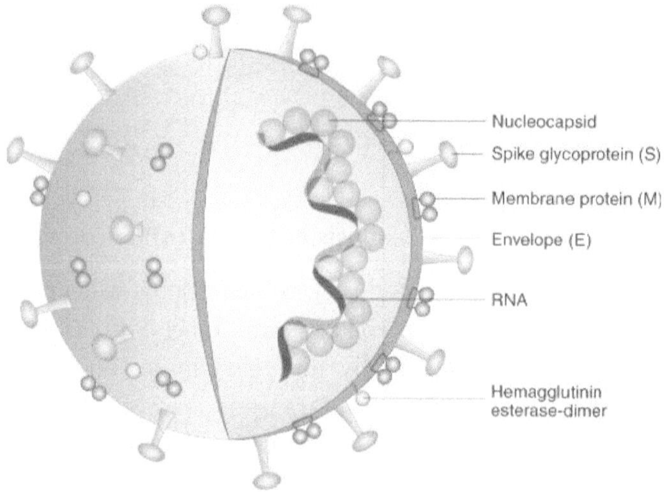

Pic 50: https://www.nature.com/articles/s41565-020-0732-3

The virus spreads primarily through respiratory droplets when infected people talk, cough, sneeze, or breathe. In crowded living conditions with poor ventilation, the virus can spread very rapidly. Large gatherings, whether for religious, social, or work purposes, have been associated with rapid spread of COVID-19.

Older adults and people with underlying health conditions like diabetes, heart disease, lung disease, or compromised immune systems are at higher risk for severe COVID-19. However, severe disease can occur in healthy people of any age.

Long-term effects of COVID-19, sometimes called "long COVID," can persist for weeks or months after the initial infection. These effects can include fatigue, shortness of breath, cognitive problems, and other symptoms that can significantly impact quality of life.

Childhood Viral Infections

Measles - The Vaccine-Preventable Danger

Measles is one of the most contagious viral infections known to humans. Before vaccines were available, nearly every child got measles, and the infection caused significant illness and death worldwide. Even today, in areas where vaccination rates are low, measles outbreaks can cause serious health problems.

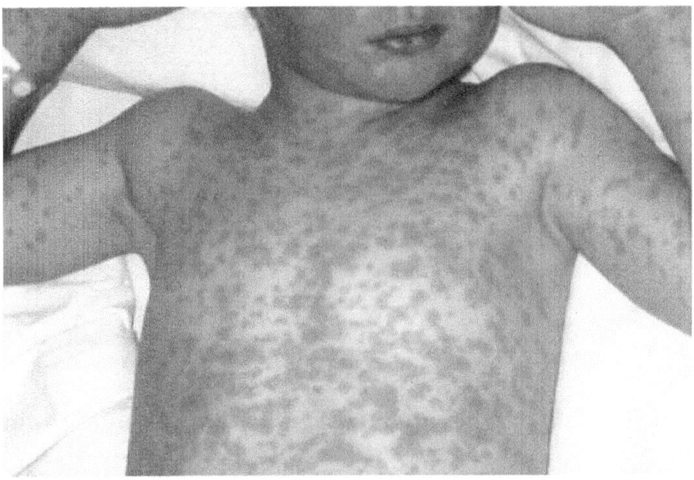

Pic 51: https:// www.webmd.com/children/vaccines/what- is-measles

The measles virus spreads through respiratory droplets and is so contagious that if one person has measles, up to 90% of nearby unvaccinated people will become infected. The virus can remain infectious in the air for up to two hours after an infected person leaves the area.

Measles typically begins with symptoms similar to a severe cold: high fever, cough, runny nose, and red, watery eyes. After a few days, a characteristic rash appears, starting on the face and spreading down the body. The rash consists of red, flat spots that may merge together as it spreads.

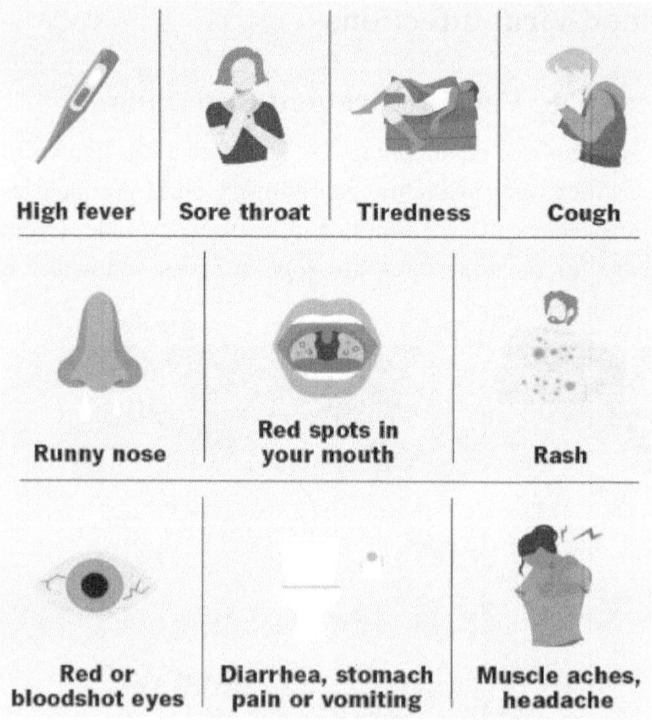

Pic 52: https://my.clevelandclinic.org/health/diseases/8584- measles

While many people recover from measles without complications, the infection can cause serious problems. Pneumonia is the most common cause of death from measles in young children. The virus can also cause brain inflammation (encephalitis), which can lead to brain damage or death.

Measles temporarily suppresses the immune system, making people more susceptible to other infections for weeks or months after recovery. This immune suppression explains why measles outbreaks are often followed by increases in other infectious diseases in affected communities.

In crowded living conditions, measles can spread extremely rapidly through families and communities. The high contagiousness of the virus means that even brief contact with an infected person can lead to transmission.

Vaccination is highly effective at preventing measles. The measles vaccine is usually given as part of the MMR (measles, mumps, rubella) vaccine. Two doses of the vaccine provide long- lasting protection against measles infection.

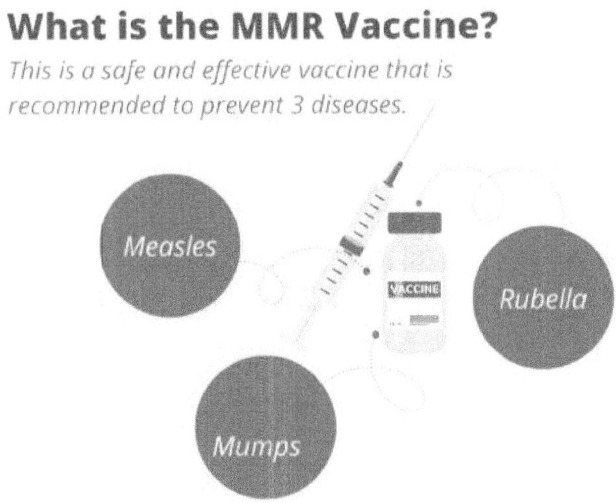

Pic 53: https://www.instagram.com/p/DOeex11kROl/

Chickenpox - The Itchy Invader

Chickenpox, caused by the varicella-zoster virus, is another common childhood viral infection that spreads easily in crowded conditions. While chickenpox is generally mild in healthy children, it can cause more serious illness in adults and people with compromised immune systems.

The hallmark of chickenpox is an itchy rash that appears as small, fluid-filled blisters all over the body. The rash typically starts on the face and chest and then spreads to other parts of the body. New blisters continue to appear for several days, so at any given time, a person with chickenpox may have blisters in different stages of development.

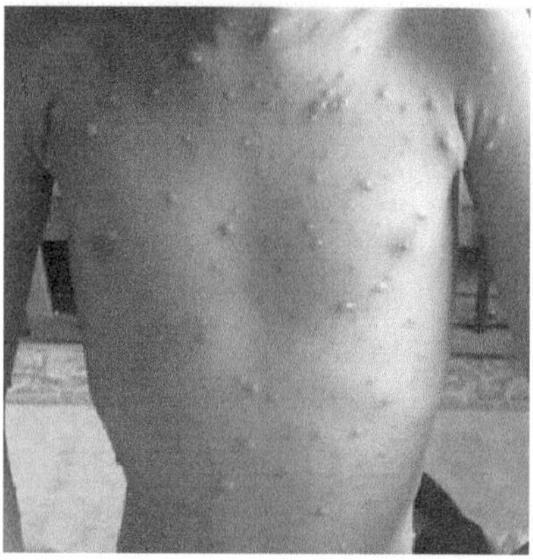

Pic 54: https://www.datelinehealthafrica.org/chickenpox-in-africans-cause-symptoms-treatment-and-prevention

Before the rash appears, people with chickenpox may have fever, headache, and fatigue. The itching from the rash can be intense and may interfere with sleep and daily activities. The blisters eventually dry up and form scabs, which fall off after one to two weeks.

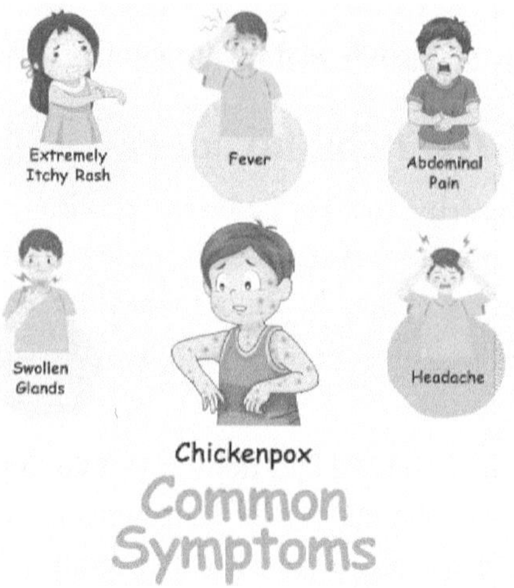
Extremely Itchy Rash
Fever
Abdominal Pain
Swollen Glands
Headache
Chickenpox
Common Symptoms

Pic 55: https://vims.ac.in/vims-hospital/

Chickenpox spreads through respiratory droplets and through direct contact with the fluid from the blisters. People with chickenpox are contagious from about two days before the rash appears until all the blisters have formed scabs.

In crowded living conditions, chickenpox can spread rapidly through families and communities, particularly affecting children who haven't been vaccinated or haven't had the infection before. Schools and daycare centers often experience outbreaks when one infected child attends while contagious.

While chickenpox is usually mild in children, complications can occur. Secondary bacterial infections of the skin are common, especially if children scratch the blisters. Pneumonia can occur, particularly in adults. Rarely, chickenpox can cause brain inflammation or other serious complications.

After a person recovers from chickenpox, the virus remains dormant in nerve cells. Later in life, usually when the immune system is weakened by aging or illness, the virus can reactivate and cause shingles, a painful condition affecting the skin and nerves.

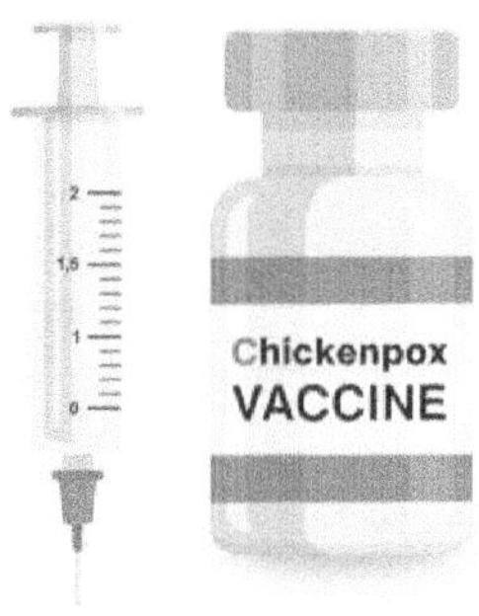

Pic 56: https://www.shutterstock.com/ Stomach Viruses - Viral Gastroenteritis

Viral gastroenteritis, often called stomach flu (though it's not related to influenza), is caused by several different types of viruses that infect the digestive system. These infections are extremely common and can affect people of all ages.

The most common viruses that cause gastroenteritis are noroviruses and rotaviruses. Noroviruses can affect people of all ages and are responsible for many outbreaks in closed communities like schools, nursing homes, and cruise ships. Rotaviruses primarily affect young children and were a leading cause of severe diarrhea in children before vaccines became available.

Symptoms of viral gastroenteritis typically include nausea, vomiting, diarrhea, stomach cramps, and sometimes fever and headache. The illness usually develops suddenly and can be quite severe for the first day or two, then gradually improves over three to seven days.

These viruses spread through the fecal-oral route, meaning that people become infected by consuming tiny amounts of contaminated material. This can happen through contaminated food or water, or by touching contaminated surfaces and then touching the mouth. Person-to-person spread can occur through close contact with infected individuals.

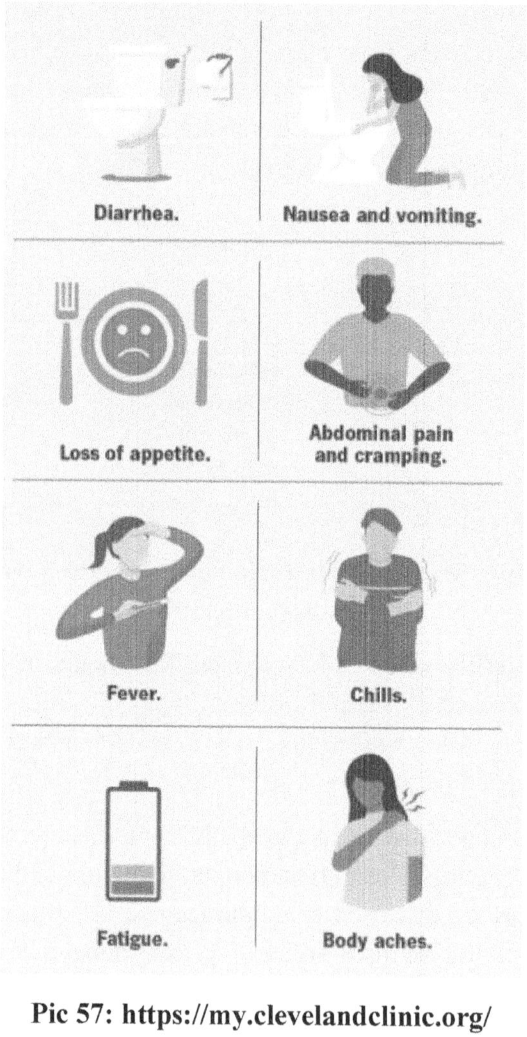

Pic 57: https://my.clevelandclinic.org/

In communities with limited access to clean water and adequate sanitation, viral gastroenteritis can spread rapidly and cause more serious illness. Dehydration from vomiting and diarrhea is the main concern, particularly in young children and elderly adults.

Crowded living conditions facilitate the spread of these viruses because they increase opportunities for person-to-person transmission and contamination of shared surfaces. Shared cooking and eating facilities can allow contaminated food or water to affect many people simultaneously.

Prevention focuses on good hygiene practices, particularly careful handwashing after using the toilet and before preparing or eating food. Access to clean water for drinking and food preparation is crucial for preventing viral gastroenteritis outbreaks.

How Your Body Fights Viruses

Natural Immune Response - Your Body's Antiviral Army

Your immune system has several specialized strategies for fighting viral infections that are different from its bacterial-fighting techniques. Understanding these antiviral defenses helps explain why viral infections often have different symptoms and recovery patterns than bacterial infections.

When viruses first enter your body, they encounter the same initial barriers that stop bacteria: skin, mucus, stomach acid, and other physical and chemical defenses. However, once viruses penetrate these barriers and begin infecting cells, your immune system must employ different tactics.

The first line of cellular defense against viruses involves interferons, special proteins that infected cells produce to warn neighboring cells about viral invasion. Interferons signal nearby cells to activate their antiviral defenses, making them more resistant to viral infection. Interferons also help activate other parts of the immune system to respond to the viral threat.

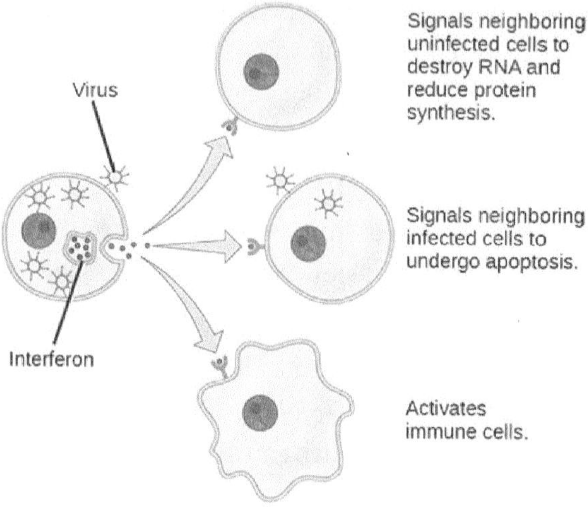

Pic 58: https://www.lecturio.com/

Natural killer cells are specialized white blood cells that can recognize and destroy virus-infected cells before the viruses have time to reproduce. These cells patrol the body looking for cells that display signs of viral infection on their surface. When they find infected cells, they inject toxic substances that kill the cell and any viruses inside it.

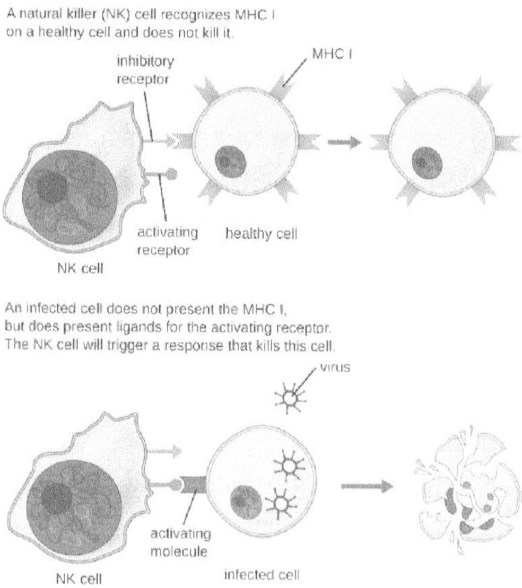

Pic 59: https://courses.lumenlearning.com/

Your immune system also produces specific antibodies designed to neutralize particular viruses. These antibodies can bind to viruses and prevent them from attaching to and infecting cells. Antibody production takes several days to weeks to reach peak levels, which explains why viral infections often get worse before they get better.

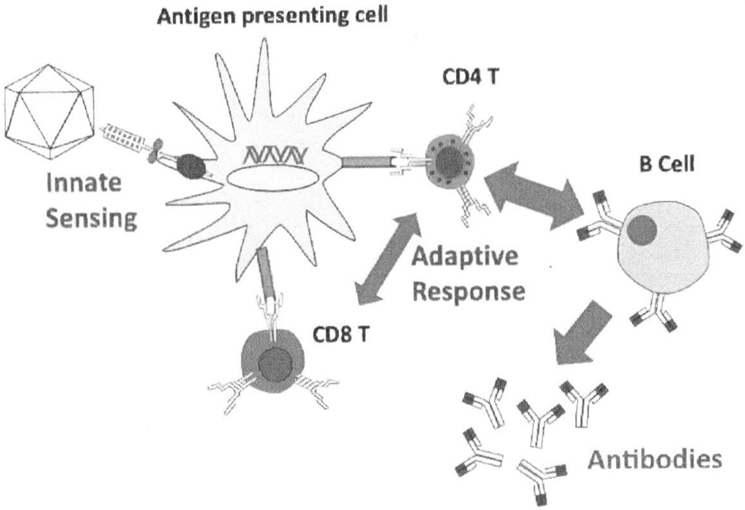

Pic 60: https://www.cell.com/ The Process:

1. **Detection**: Your body has special "guard cells" (the Antigen Presenting Cell in the center) that patrol and detect when something harmful enters your body, like bacteria or viruses.
2. **Alert System**: When these guard cells find something dangerous, they grab pieces of it and show it to your "commander cells" (the CD4 T and CD8 T cells). This is like showing a wanted poster to security guards.
3. **Calling for Backup**: The commander cells then send signals to your "factory cells" (B cells - the blue cell on the right) telling them exactly what to make to fight the specific threat.
4. **Making Weapons**: The factory cells (B cells) then produce special weapons called antibodies (the Y- shaped things at the bottom) that are custom-designed to attack and neutralize that specific threat.

Memory cells are perhaps the most important component of antiviral immunity. After your immune system successfully fights off a viral infection, it retains specialized memory cells that remember the specific virus. If you encounter the same virus again, these memory cells can quickly organize a defense, often preventing illness entirely or reducing its severity.

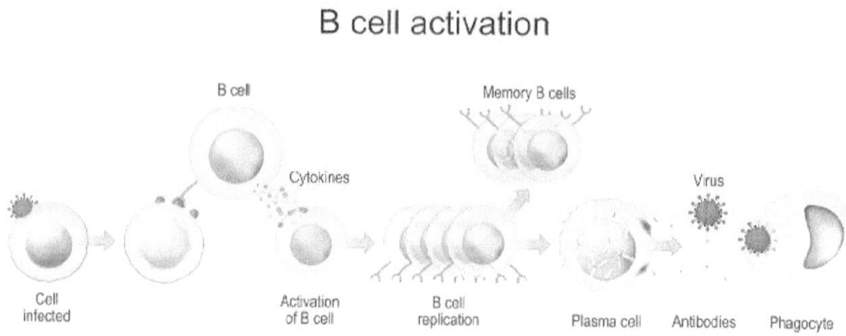

Pic 61: https://www.dreamstime.com/

Why Rest and Fluids Help - Supporting Your Immune System

Supporting your immune system during viral infections is crucial because your body must do most of the work of eliminating the virus. Unlike bacterial infections, which can often be cured with antibiotics, viral infections usually require your immune system to clear the virus naturally.

Rest is essential during viral infections because fighting viruses requires significant energy. When you're active, your body's energy is divided between normal activities and immune function. Resting allows your body to dedicate more resources to producing immune cells, antibodies, and other infection- fighting substances.

During sleep, your body produces higher levels of certain immune cells and antibodies. Sleep also helps regulate the production of stress hormones that can suppress immune function. People who don't get adequate rest during viral infections often experience longer illness duration and more severe symptoms.

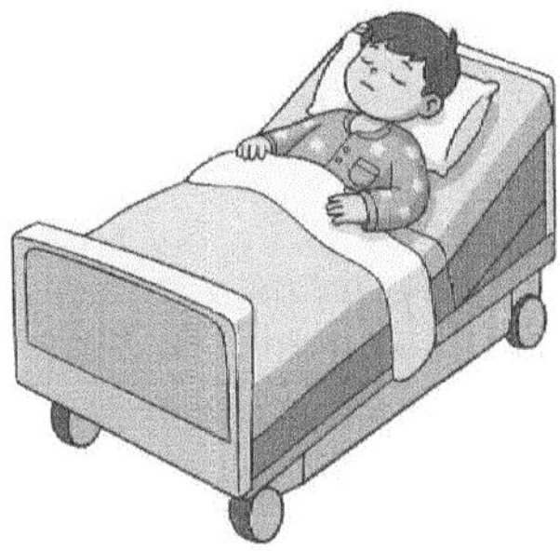

Pic 62: https://www.vectorstock.com/

Adequate fluid intake is crucial during viral infections for several reasons. Fever, which commonly accompanies viral infections, increases fluid losses through sweating and breathing. Dehydration can impair immune function and make it harder for your body to fight the infection.

Fluids also help maintain the moisture of mucous membranes in the nose and throat. These membranes are important barriers against viral invasion, and they function better when properly hydrated. Adequate hydration also helps the kidneys eliminate waste products produced during the immune response.

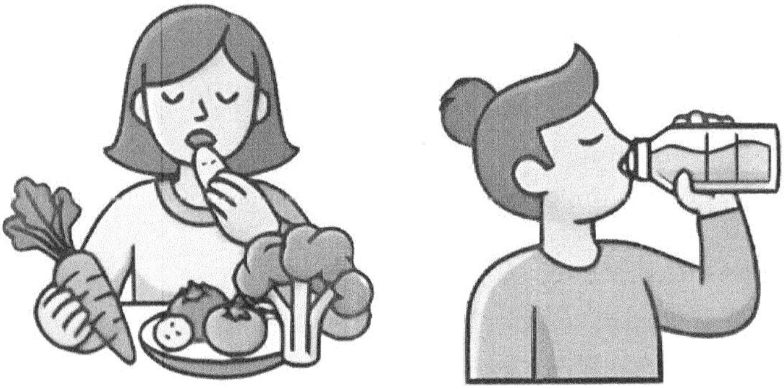

Pic 63: https://www.dreamstime.com/

Good nutrition supports immune function during viral infections, though appetite is often reduced when people are sick. Protein is particularly important because immune cells and antibodies are made primarily of protein. Vitamins and minerals also play crucial roles in immune function.

Symptom management can make viral infections more tolerable while the immune system does its work. Fever reducers like acetaminophen or ibuprofen can help with discomfort, though low-grade fever actually helps the immune system fight infection. Pain relievers can help with headaches and muscle aches.

For respiratory viral infections, humidified air can help soothe irritated airways and make breathing more comfortable. Steam from hot showers or bowls of hot water can provide temporary relief. Saline nasal rinses can help clear congestion.

Antiviral medications are available for some viral infections, though they are much less common than antibiotics. These medicines work by interfering with specific steps in viral reproduction. Examples include oseltamivir (Tamiflu) for influenza and acyclovir for herpes infections.

Antiviral medications are most effective when started early in the course of infection, often within 48 hours of symptom onset. They typically reduce the duration and severity of illness rather than providing immediate cures like many antibiotics do for bacterial infections.

How Antiviral Drugs Work

Entry and Early Stage Inhibition

Entry Inhibition: Drugs block viruses from attaching to or entering host cells by targeting viral surface proteins or cellular receptors.

Uncoating Inhibition: Once inside, some drugs prevent the virus from releasing its genetic material into the cell.

Replication Interference

Reverse Transcriptase & RNase-H Inhibition: Particularly important for retroviruses like HIV, these drugs block enzymes that convert viral RNA into DNA.

Viral Polymerase Inhibition: Drugs interfere with viral enzymes responsible for copying viral genetic material (DNA or RNA).

Chain Termination: Some drugs get incorporated into growing viral DNA/RNA chains, causing premature termination of replication.

Nucleotide Synthesis Inhibition: Drugs block the production of building blocks (nucleotides) needed for viral genetic material.

Integration and Protein Processing

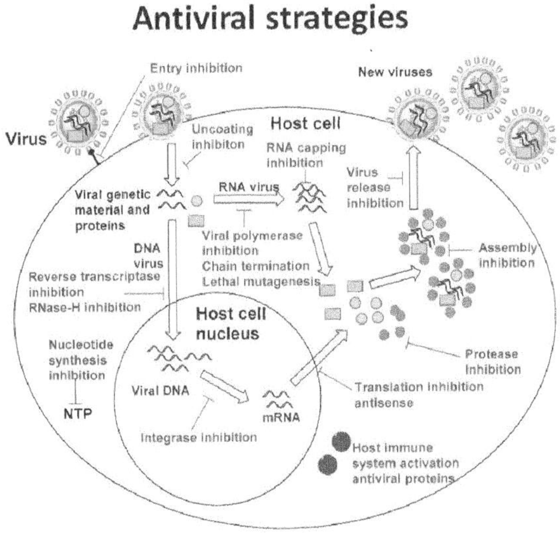

Pic 64: https://www.mdpi.com/1999-4915/13/4/667

Integrase Inhibition: Prevents viral DNA from integrating into the host cell's genome (crucial for HIV treatment).

Protease Inhibition: Blocks viral enzymes that cut newly made viral proteins into their functional forms.

Translation Inhibition: Antisense drugs interfere with the production of viral proteins.

Assembly and Release

Assembly Inhibition: Prevents newly made viral components from assembling into complete virus particles.

Virus Release Inhibition: Blocks mature viruses from leaving the host cell to infect other cells.

Host Defense Enhancement

Host Immune System Activation: Some drugs boost the body's natural antiviral defenses rather than directly targeting the virus.

Recovery Timeline - How Long Viral Infections Usually Last

Understanding the typical timeline of viral infections helps people know what to expect and when to seek additional medical care. Most viral infections follow predictable patterns, though the exact duration can vary based on the specific virus, the person's immune system, and other factors.

Most viral infections have an incubation period between exposure and symptom development. This period can range from one to fourteen days, depending on the virus. During this time, the virus is multiplying in the body, but symptoms haven't yet appeared.

The acute phase of viral illness, when symptoms are most severe, typically lasts three to seven days for most common viral infections. During this phase, the immune system is actively fighting the virus, which causes most of the symptoms people experience.

Recovery from viral infections is usually gradual. Symptoms slowly improve over one to two weeks as the immune system gains control over the viral infection. Some symptoms, particularly fatigue, may persist for weeks after other symptoms have resolved.

Certain viral infections have longer recovery periods. Mononucleosis, caused by the Epstein-Barr virus, can cause fatigue that lasts for months. Some people experience prolonged symptoms after COVID-19 infection. These extended recovery periods usually occur because the virus has caused more extensive tissue damage or because the immune response has been particularly intense.

Why Antibiotics Don't Work on Viruses Different Targets - Bacteria vs. Virus Structure

The fundamental reason antibiotics don't work against viruses lies in the completely different structures and life processes of bacteria versus viruses. Antibiotics are designed to target specific features of bacterial cells that are not present in viruses or human cells.

Antibiotics have no effect on viral infections. Viruses have completely different structures and reproduction mechanisms than bacteria, so medicines designed to kill bacteria cannot kill viruses. Taking antibiotics for viral infections like the common cold or flu will not help recovery and may cause unnecessary side effects.

Even for bacterial infections, not all antibiotics work against all bacteria. Bacteria have developed many different resistance mechanisms that can make them immune to certain antibiotics. Using the wrong antibiotic for a particular bacterial infection may be ineffective, allowing the infection to continue or worsen.

Some bacteria have natural resistance to certain antibiotics. Other bacteria may acquire resistance through genetic changes or by obtaining resistance genes from other bacteria. Antibiotic resistance can develop in individual patients during treatment if antibiotics are not used properly.

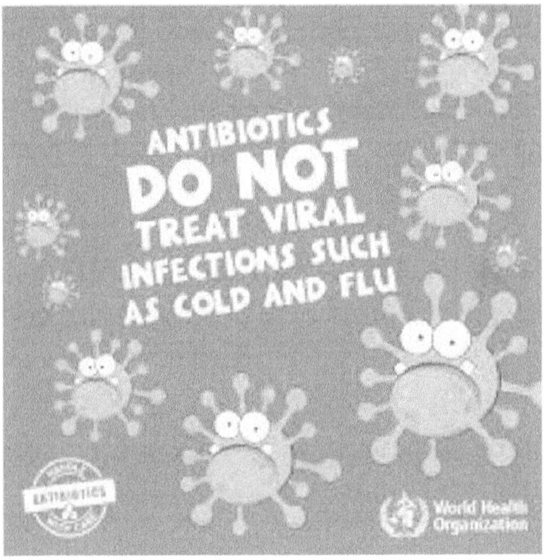
ANTIBIOTICS
DO NOT
TREAT VIRAL
INFECTIONS SUCH
AS COLD AND FLU
World Health
Organization

Pic 65: https://www.facebook.com/WHO

Taking antibiotics when they are not needed can harm the beneficial bacteria that normally live in and on your body. These good bacteria help protect against infection and support various body functions. When antibiotics kill these protective bacteria, harmful bacteria may be able to take their place.

Some antibiotics work by interfering with bacterial metabolism - the chemical processes that bacteria use to generate energy and build cellular components. Viruses don't have their own metabolism; they rely entirely on the host cell's metabolic processes. Therefore, antibiotics that disrupt bacterial metabolism have no effect on viruses.

Community Focus: Preventing Viral Spread or Crowded Conditions

Why Viruses Spread Faster in Slums

Viral infections spread more rapidly in crowded living conditions for several interconnected reasons that create ideal environments for transmission. Understanding these factors helps communities develop strategies to reduce viral spread even when living conditions cannot be immediately changed.

Physical proximity is the most obvious factor that increases viral transmission. When many people live in small spaces, they have frequent close contact with each other, increasing opportunities for viruses to jump from person to person through respiratory droplets, direct contact, or contaminated surfaces.

Shared living spaces mean that when one person becomes infected, they can easily expose many others before they realize they're sick. Family members sharing beds or sleeping areas have particularly high risk of transmission, especially for respiratory viruses that spread through droplets and airborne particles.

Limited access to isolation spaces makes it difficult to separate sick family members from healthy ones. When someone develops a viral infection, they may continue to share living spaces, cooking areas, and bathroom facilities with others, providing ongoing opportunities for transmission.

High population density also means that viral outbreaks can affect large numbers of people quickly. When infections spread rapidly through a community, healthcare resources can become overwhelmed, making it harder to provide appropriate care for those who need it.

Economic factors often force people to continue working or going to school even when they're mildly ill, further spreading viruses throughout the community. The inability to take time off work for illness creates a cycle where infections continue to spread.

Ventilation Importance - Fresh Air as Prevention

Good ventilation is one of the most effective ways to reduce the spread of respiratory viruses, yet it's often lacking in crowded living conditions. Understanding how ventilation works helps communities find ways to improve air circulation even with limited resources.

When people breathe, talk, cough, or sneeze, they release tiny droplets and aerosols that can contain viruses. In poorly ventilated spaces, these infectious particles can remain suspended in the air for hours, increasing the chance that other people will breathe them in.

Good ventilation works by diluting the concentration of viral particles in the air and by removing contaminated air from living spaces. Fresh air from outside typically contains no infectious particles, so increasing the amount of outside air that enters living spaces reduces viral transmission risk.

Natural ventilation through open windows and doors can significantly improve air quality in homes and community buildings. Even opening windows partially can increase air circulation. Cross-ventilation, created by opening windows or doors on opposite sides of a room, is particularly effective.

In areas where opening windows isn't possible due to weather, security, or other concerns, fans can help improve air circulation. Fans that blow air out of windows help remove contaminated air from inside spaces. Ceiling fans or portable fans can help keep air moving, though they don't remove contaminated air from the space.

Community buildings like schools, religious centers, and meeting halls should prioritize ventilation improvements. These spaces often have large numbers of people in close proximity, creating high-risk environments for viral transmission.

Isolation When Possible - Protecting Family Members

While complete isolation may not be possible in crowded living conditions, even partial separation of sick family members can significantly reduce viral transmission to others. Creative approaches to isolation can be effective even in small spaces.

Creating physical barriers within shared spaces can help reduce transmission. Hanging sheets or curtains can provide some separation between sick and healthy family members. Keeping sick family members in one area of the home as much as possible reduces the number of surfaces and areas that become contaminated.

Timing strategies can also provide some protection. Having sick family members eat meals at different times or use bathroom facilities at different times can reduce exposure opportunities. Scheduling activities so that sick and healthy family members are in shared spaces at different times provides some protection.

Sick family members should sleep separately when possible, even if this means sleeping on floors or other less comfortable arrangements temporarily. Respiratory viruses spread easily during sleep through breathing and coughing, so shared sleeping spaces create high transmission risk.

When complete isolation isn't possible, sick family members should try to maintain distance from others and wear masks or cover their faces when coughing or sneezing. Simple cloth face coverings can significantly reduce the number of infectious droplets released into the air.

Designating specific items for use by sick family members can help prevent contamination of shared objects. Having separate eating utensils, towels, and personal items for sick family members reduces transmission through contaminated surfaces.

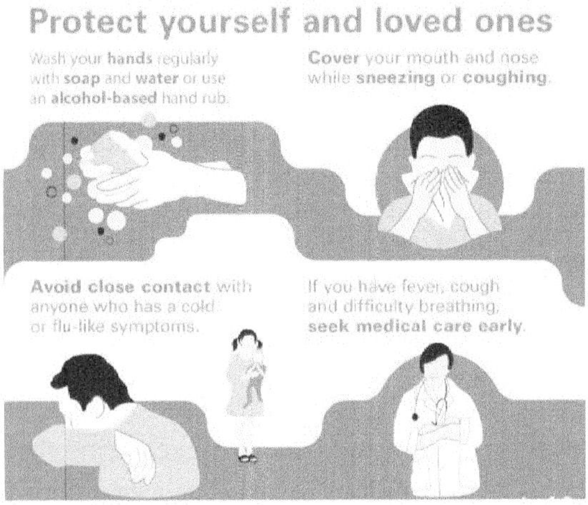
Protect yourself and loved ones
Wash your hands regularly with soap and water or use an alcohol-based hand rub.
Cover your mouth and nose while sneezing or coughing.
Avoid close contact with anyone who has a cold or flu-like symptoms.
If you have fever, cough and difficulty breathing, seek medical care early.

Pic 66: https://www.unicef.org/

Hygiene Practices - Hand Washing, Covering Coughs

Basic hygiene practices remain the most effective and accessible methods for preventing viral transmission in any community. These practices are particularly important in crowded conditions where transmission opportunities are frequent.

Hand washing is the single most important hygiene practice for preventing viral infections. Hands become contaminated when people touch infected surfaces or when respiratory droplets land on them. Regular, thorough hand washing removes viruses before they can be transferred to the mouth, nose, or eyes.

Effective hand washing requires soap and water and should last at least 20 seconds. All surfaces of the hands should be scrubbed, including between fingers, under nails, and around wrists. When soap and water aren't available, alcohol-based hand sanitizers with at least 60% alcohol content can provide some protection.

Hand washing should occur frequently throughout the day, particularly before eating, after using the toilet, after coughing or sneezing, after touching shared surfaces, and after caring for sick family members. In crowded conditions, hands should be washed more frequently because contamination opportunities are more common.

Covering coughs and sneezes prevents the release of infectious droplets into the air where others can breathe them in. The best technique is to cough or sneeze into the elbow rather than into hands, since hands are more likely to touch other surfaces and spread contamination.

When tissues are available, they should be used once and then disposed of immediately. Hands should be washed after disposing of used tissues. Used tissues should be kept away from other family members and disposed of in ways that don't create contamination.

Avoiding touching the face, particularly the mouth, nose, and eyes, prevents viruses on contaminated hands from entering the body. This can be challenging because people touch their faces frequently throughout the day, often without realizing it.

Chapter - 7
Parasites and Fungi - The Freeloaders

"Other unwanted guests"

Parasites: Living Off Your Body

Intestinal Worms

How You Get Them - Contaminated Food, Water, and Soil

Intestinal worms are among the most common parasitic infections worldwide, affecting billions of people, particularly in communities with limited access to clean water and adequate sanitation. These parasites have complex life cycles that often involve contaminated soil, water, or food, making them particularly common in areas where human waste management is inadequate.

The most common intestinal worms include roundworms, hookworms, whipworms, and tapeworms. Each type has a different method of entering the human body, but all share the characteristic of living in the intestines where they feed on nutrients intended for their human host.

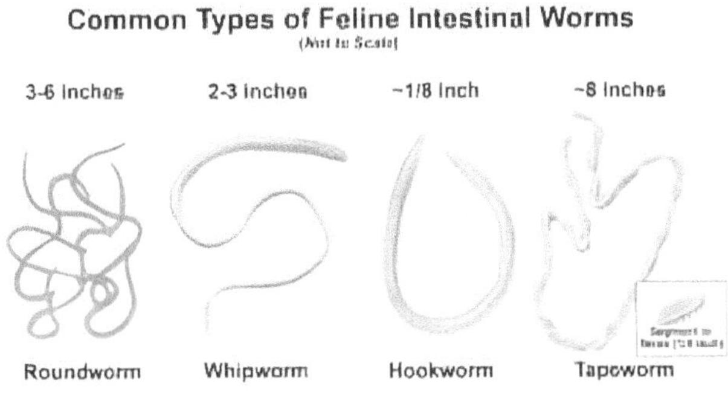

Pic 67: https://www.npvet.co.nz/

Roundworm infections typically occur when people consume food or water contaminated with roundworm eggs. These microscopic eggs can survive in soil for years, waiting for the opportunity to enter a human host. When vegetables are grown in contaminated soil and not properly washed, or when water sources are contaminated with human waste, roundworm eggs can easily be consumed.

Hookworm infections often occur when people walk barefoot on soil contaminated with hookworm larvae. The tiny larvae can penetrate through the skin of the feet and then travel through the bloodstream to the lungs, where they are coughed up and swallowed, finally reaching the intestines where they mature into adult worms.

Tapeworm infections usually result from eating undercooked meat from infected animals. Pork, beef, and fish can all harbour tapeworm larvae in their muscles. When this meat is not cooked to temperatures hot enough to kill the larvae, people can become infected by consuming the parasites.

Poor sanitation creates ideal conditions for worm transmission. When human waste is not properly disposed of, worm eggs and larvae can contaminate soil and water sources. In areas without adequate toilet facilities, people may defecate in areas where others walk, work, or play, creating ongoing cycles of contamination and reinfection.

Crowded living conditions increase the risk of worm infections because they often coincide with poor sanitation and because infected family members can easily transmit certain types of worms to others. Some worms, like pinworms, can spread directly from person to person through contaminated hands and surfaces.

Signs You Have Them - Stomach Pain, Weight Loss

Intestinal worm infections can cause a wide range of symptoms, though some people may have no symptoms at all, especially in the early stages of infection. Learning to recognize the signs of worm infections helps people seek appropriate treatment before complications develop.

Stomach pain and digestive problems are among the most common symptoms of intestinal worms. This pain may be constant or intermittent and can range from mild discomfort to severe cramping. The location of the pain may vary depending on where in the intestines the worms are living.

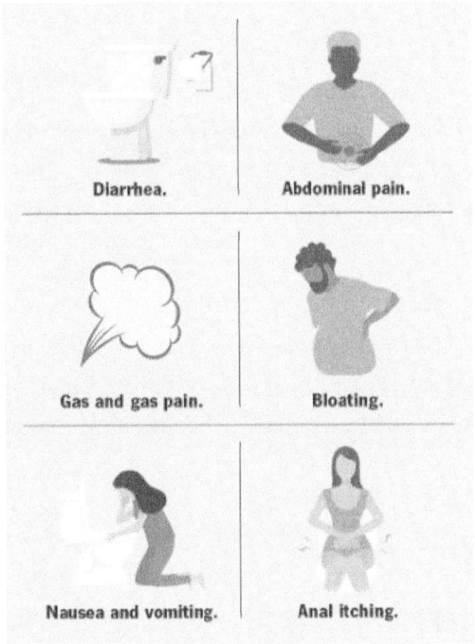

Pic 68: https://my.clevelandclinic.org/

Changes in bowel movements often occur with worm infections. Some people develop diarrhea, while others experience constipation. The stool may contain blood or mucus, particularly with certain types of worm infections. In some cases, people may actually see worms or worm segments in their stool.

Unexplained weight loss despite normal or increased appetite is a significant sign of intestinal worm infection. The worms consume nutrients that should nourish the human host, leading to malnutrition even when people are eating adequate amounts of food. Children with chronic worm infections may fail to grow and develop normally.

Fatigue and weakness often develop as worm infections progress. This occurs partly because the worms are consuming nutrients and partly because some worms cause blood loss, leading to anemia. People may feel tired even after adequate rest and may have difficulty concentrating or performing normal activities.

Changes in appetite can occur with worm infections. Some people lose their appetite entirely, while others develop unusual cravings or feel hungry all the time despite eating. Nausea and vomiting may also occur, particularly if the worm burden is heavy.

In children, behavioral changes may be noticed. Infected children may become irritable, have difficulty sleeping, or experience changes in school performance. Some children may develop the habit of grinding their teeth, especially at night, though this symptom can have many causes.

Visible signs may sometimes appear. With hookworm infections, people may notice itchy, red tracks on their skin where the larvae entered. Some worm infections can cause a swollen belly, particularly in children. Pinworm infections often cause intense itching around the anus, especially at night.

Community Treatment Approaches

Treating intestinal worm infections effectively often requires community-wide approaches rather than just treating individual cases. This is because the environmental conditions that allow worms to spread typically affect entire communities, and reinfection can occur quickly if these conditions aren't addressed.

Mass drug administration programs, where entire communities receive anti-worm medications regardless of whether they have symptoms, can be highly effective in areas where worm infections are common. These programs treat everyone simultaneously, reducing the overall number of worms in the community and breaking transmission cycles.

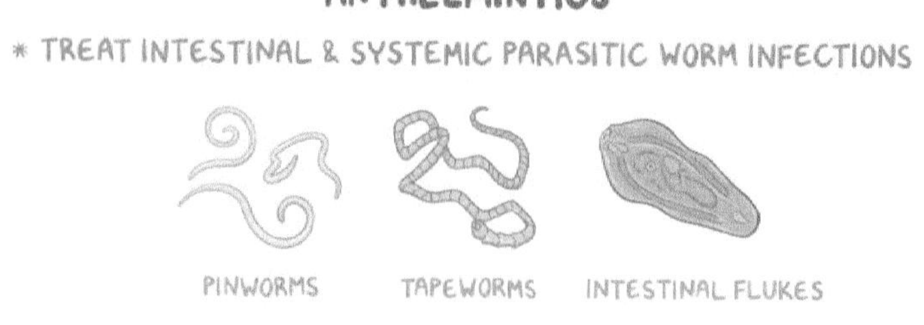

Pic 69: https://www.osmosis.org/

The medications used to treat worm infections, called anthelmintics, are generally safe and effective. Different medications work against different types of worms, so proper diagnosis helps ensure the right treatment is used. In community programs, broad-spectrum medications that work against multiple types of worms are often used.

However, medication alone is not sufficient for long-term control of worm infections. Environmental improvements are essential for preventing reinfection. This includes improving sanitation facilities, ensuring access to clean water, and educating communities about hygiene practices.

Community education plays a crucial role in worm prevention and control. Teaching people about how worms spread, how to recognize symptoms, and how to prevent infection helps reduce transmission. This education should be culturally appropriate and delivered in languages and formats that community members can understand.

Regular deworming programs in schools can be particularly effective because children are often at higher risk for worm infections and can serve as sources of transmission to their families. School-based programs also provide opportunities to teach children about hygiene and prevention.

Blood Parasites

Malaria - The Mosquito-Transmitted Killer

Malaria remains one of the world's most serious parasitic diseases, causing hundreds of thousands of deaths annually, particularly among children in sub-Saharan Africa. Understanding malaria transmission, symptoms, and prevention is crucial for communities in areas where the disease is common.

Malaria is caused by parasites called Plasmodium, which are transmitted to humans through the bites of infected female Anopheles mosquitoes. There are several species of malaria parasites, with Plasmodium falciparum being the most dangerous and most likely to cause severe disease and death.

The malaria transmission cycle is complex and involves both humans and mosquitoes. When an infected mosquito bites a human, it injects malaria parasites into the bloodstream. These parasites travel to the liver, where they multiply and mature. After several days or weeks, the parasites leave the liver and enter red blood cells, where they continue to multiply.

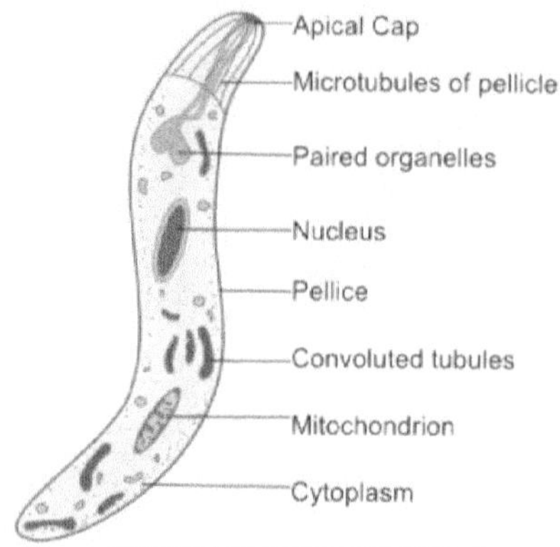

Pic 70: https://www.studyandscore.com/

As the parasites reproduce inside red blood cells, they eventually cause the cells to burst, releasing more parasites into the bloodstream. This cyclical destruction of red blood cells causes the characteristic symptoms of malaria and can lead to severe anemia if untreated.

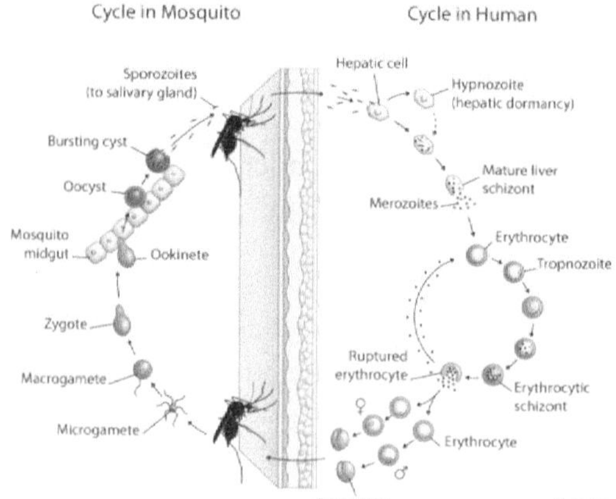

Pic 71: http://www.malwest.gr/en-us

When a mosquito bites a person infected with malaria, it ingests the parasites along with blood. The parasites then develop inside the mosquito for about two weeks before the mosquito becomes capable of transmitting malaria to other people through subsequent bites.

Environmental factors greatly influence malaria transmission. Anopheles mosquitoes require standing water to lay their eggs and complete their life cycle. Poor drainage, water storage containers, and seasonal flooding can create ideal breeding conditions for these mosquitoes.

Climate also affects malaria transmission. Warmer temperatures allow both mosquitoes and parasites to develop more quickly, potentially increasing transmission rates. Rainfall patterns influence mosquito breeding opportunities and can affect the timing and intensity of malaria seasons.

Recognition and Rapid Treatment Importance

Early recognition and prompt treatment of malaria are crucial for preventing severe complications and death. Malaria symptoms can develop rapidly, particularly with Plasmodium falciparum infections, making quick diagnosis and treatment essential.

The classic symptoms of malaria include fever, chills, and sweating, often occurring in cyclical patterns that correspond to the parasite's life cycle in red blood cells. However, early malaria symptoms can be quite general and may resemble many other illnesses, including flu, making diagnosis challenging.

Fever is the most common symptom of malaria and may be the only early sign. The fever may be constant or may come and go in patterns. Some people experience severe chills followed by high fever and then profuse sweating as the fever breaks. However, not all malaria cases follow this classic pattern.

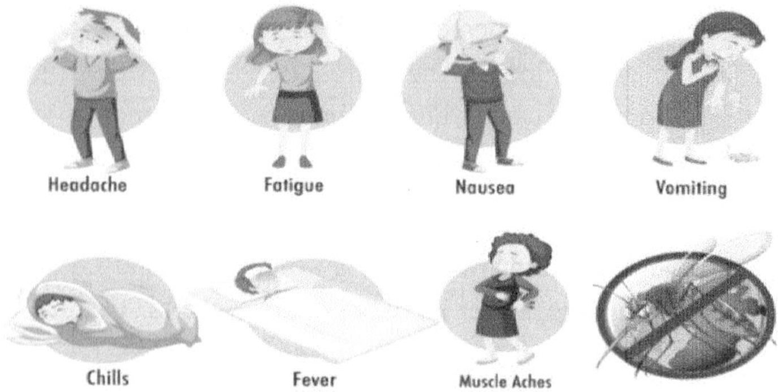

Pic 72: https://www.aimsindia.com/

Other common symptoms include headache, muscle aches, fatigue, nausea, and vomiting. These symptoms can be mild initially but may worsen rapidly, particularly with falciparum malaria. Children may develop additional symptoms like irritability, poor feeding, or unusual sleepiness.

Severe malaria can develop within hours in some cases, particularly in children, pregnant women, and people with no previous exposure to malaria. Signs of severe malaria include difficulty breathing, confusion or loss of consciousness, seizures, severe anemia, and kidney failure.

The importance of rapid treatment cannot be overstated. Delays in treatment, even of just a few hours, can mean the difference between mild illness and life-threatening complications. In areas where malaria is common, any fever should be considered malaria until proven otherwise.

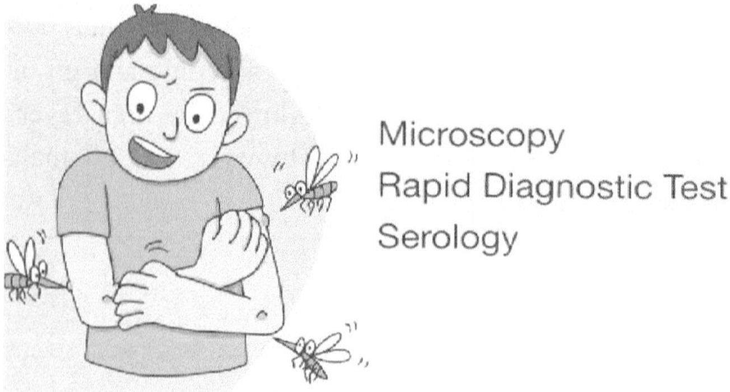

Pic 73: https://www.pacehospital.com/malaria-symptoms-causes

Rapid diagnostic tests for malaria have made it possible to diagnose the disease quickly even in remote areas without laboratory facilities. These tests can detect malaria parasites in a drop of blood within 15-20 minutes, allowing treatment to begin immediately.

How is malaria treated?

Antimalarial medications can treat malaria and clear the infection from your body, but it's important to start treatment as soon as possible. If malaria isn't treated properly, it can cause serious health problems, including permanent organ damage and death. Your provider will prescribe medications to kill the type of *Plasmodium* parasite responsible for your infection. Some parasites are resistant to malaria drugs.

Antimalarial drugs include: Atovaquone, Chloroquine, Doxycycline, Mefloquine, Quinine, Primaquine etc

Vaccine against malaria?

Two vaccines that help protect against malaria are available. Public health officials recommend vaccination against malaria for children who live in areas where infections are common.

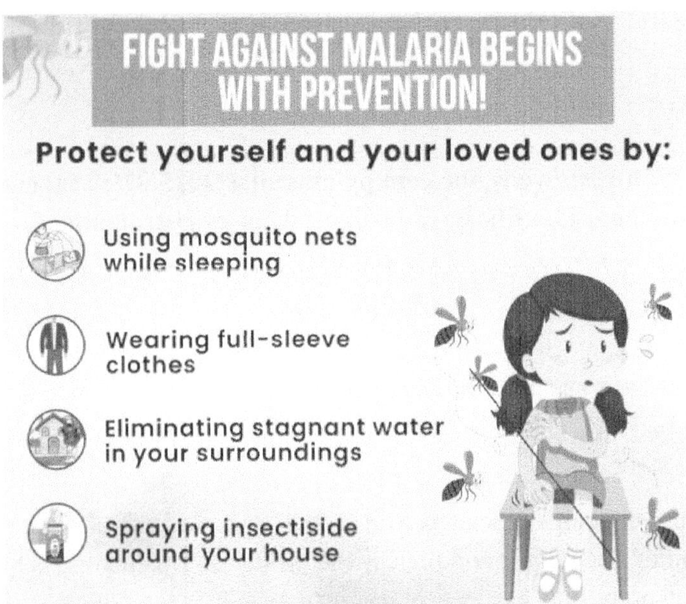

Pic 74: https://x.com/MoHFW_INDIA

External Parasites

Scabies - The Itchy Skin Mites

Scabies is a highly contagious skin infestation caused by tiny mites called Sarcoptes scabiei. These microscopic parasites burrow into the outer layer of human skin, where they live and reproduce, causing intense itching and skin irritation.

The scabies mite is incredibly small, about the size of a pinhead, and cannot be seen with the naked eye. Female mites burrow into the skin and create tunnels where they lay their eggs. These tunnels appear as thin, wavy lines on the skin surface and are most commonly found between fingers, on wrists, elbows, armpits, waist, and genital areas.

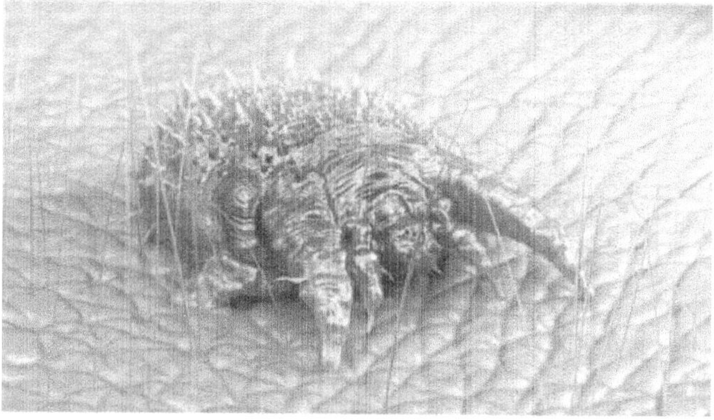

Pic75: https://www.abc.com.py/mascotas/2025/07/30/sarna-en-perros-como-identificar-cada-tipo-y-cual-es-el-tratamiento- mas-efectivo/

Scabies spreads through prolonged, direct skin-to-skin contact with an infected person. Brief contact, such as shaking hands, is usually not sufficient for transmission. However, the mites can also spread through sharing bedding, clothing, or towels with an infected person, though this is less common.

The intense itching associated with scabies is actually an allergic reaction to the mites, their eggs, and their waste products. This itching is typically worse at night and can be so severe that it interferes with sleep. The itching may continue for several weeks even after successful treatment because it takes time for the allergic reaction to subside.

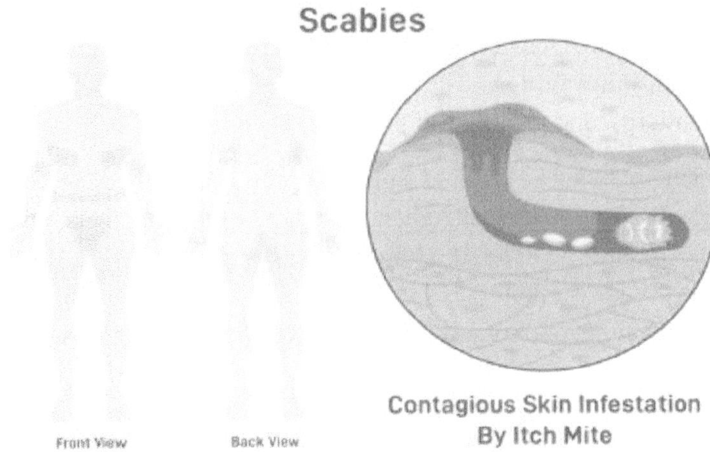

Pic 76: https://www.123rf.com/photo_194474401_scabies-skin-infestation-with-itch-mite-infected-microscopic- epidermis.html

In crowded living conditions, scabies can spread rapidly through families and communities. Children are particularly susceptible because they often have close physical contact with others. Shared sleeping arrangements and limited access to clean clothing and bedding facilitate transmission.

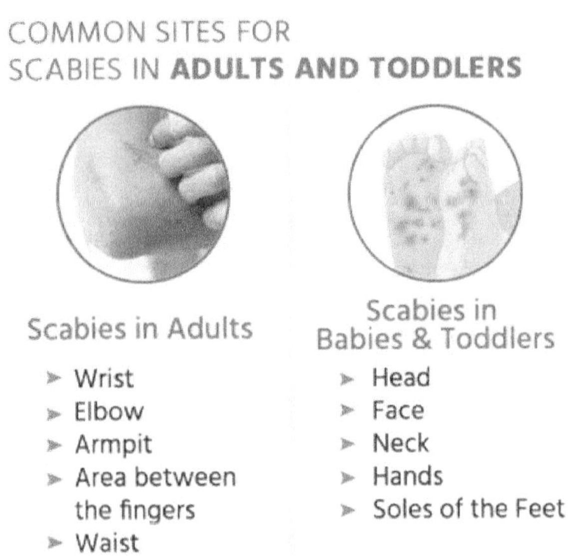

Pic 77: https://www.medicoverhospitals.in/diseases/scabies/

The diagnosis of scabies is usually made based on the characteristic itching and skin changes, along with a history of possible exposure. Sometimes, mites or eggs can be identified by examining skin scrapings under a microscope, but this is not always necessary for diagnosis.

Treatment for scabies involves applying prescription medications to the entire body from the neck down. All household members and close contacts should be treated simultaneously, even if they don't have symptoms, because they may be infected but not yet showing signs. All clothing, bedding, and towels should be washed in hot water and dried in a hot dryer.

Head Lice - The Social Spreaders

Head lice are small, wingless insects that live on the human scalp and feed on blood. While head lice don't transmit diseases, they are highly contagious and can spread rapidly through communities, particularly affecting school-age children.

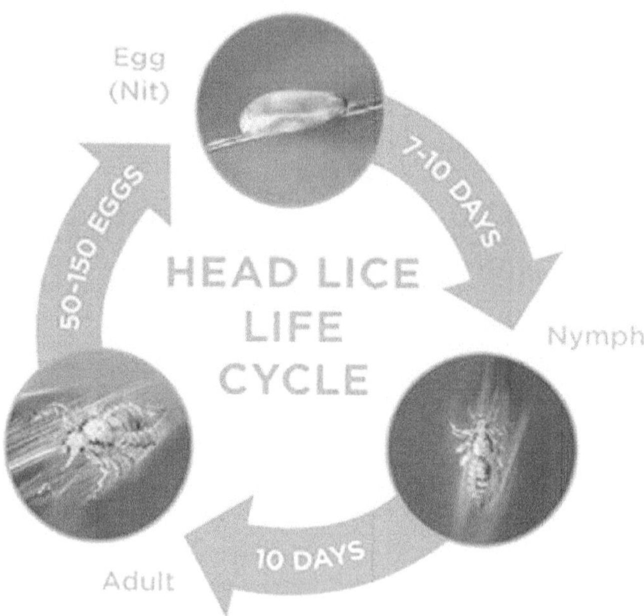

Pic 78: https://www.liceclinics.gr/en/lice-facts/

Adult head lice are about the size of a sesame seed and are brown or grayish in color. They have six legs with claws that allow them to grasp tightly to hair strands. Lice eggs, called nits, are attached to hair shafts close to the scalp and appear as small, oval-shaped specks that may be white, yellow, or brown.

Head lice spread primarily through direct head-to-head contact. They cannot jump or fly but can crawl quickly from one head to another when people's heads touch. This type of contact is common among children during play, sports activities, or when sharing personal items.

While less common, head lice can also spread through sharing personal items that come into contact with the head, such as hats, helmets, hair brushes, or headphones. However, lice cannot survive for more than 24-48 hours away from the human scalp, so transmission through objects is relatively uncommon.

The most common symptom of head lice is itching, caused by an allergic reaction to lice saliva. However, not everyone with head lice experiences itching, and some people may have lice for weeks before noticing any symptoms. Scratching can lead to secondary bacterial infections of the scalp.

Diagnosing head lice requires careful examination of the hair and scalp. Live lice are often difficult to find because they move quickly and avoid light. Nits are easier to spot and are usually found within a quarter-inch of the scalp. Empty nit shells may remain attached to hair shafts even after lice have been eliminated.

Treatment for head lice involves using medicated shampoos or lotions specifically designed to kill lice and nits. Multiple treatments are usually necessary because no product is 100% effective at killing all nits, and new lice may hatch from surviving eggs.

In communities where head lice are common, preventing spread requires community-wide awareness and cooperation. Schools and childcare centers should have policies for checking children and managing outbreaks. Teaching children not to share personal items that touch the head helps reduce transmission.

Fungi: The Moisture Lovers

Skin Fungal Infections

Athlete's Foot - Between the Toes

Athlete's foot is one of the most common fungal infections affecting humans, caused by fungi that thrive in warm, moist environments. Despite its name, athlete's foot can affect anyone and is particularly common in communities where people share bathing facilities or walk barefoot in contaminated areas.

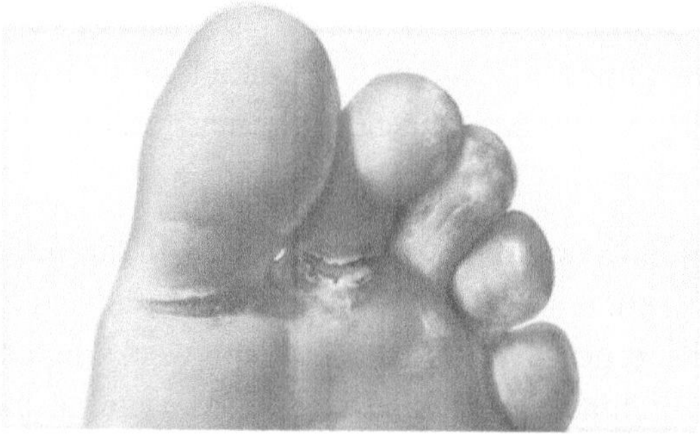

Pic 79: https://kidshealth.org/en/teens/athletes-foot.html

The fungi that cause athlete's foot belong to a group called dermatophytes (*Trichophyton)*, which specialize in infecting skin, hair, and nails. These fungi produce enzymes that break down keratin, the protein that makes up the outer layer of skin, allowing them to penetrate and establish infections.

Athlete's foot typically affects the spaces between the toes, particularly between the fourth and fifth toes where moisture tends to accumulate. The infection causes the skin to become red, itchy, and scaly. In severe cases, the skin may crack or blister, creating openings for bacterial infections.

The fungi that cause athlete's foot are found naturally in the environment and can survive for long periods on surfaces like bathroom floors, shower stalls, and pool areas. People become infected when they walk barefoot in these contaminated areas and the fungi find suitable conditions on their feet.

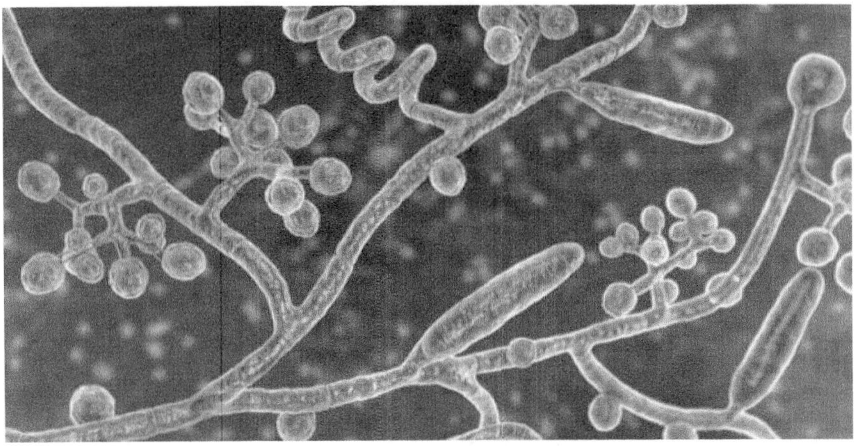

Pic 80: https://www.shutterstock.com/

Warm, moist conditions create ideal environments for fungal growth. Feet that are kept in closed shoes for long periods, especially without adequate ventilation, provide perfect conditions for athlete's foot to develop. Synthetic materials that don't allow feet to breathe increase the risk of infection.

Sweaty feet, poor foot hygiene, and shared bathing facilities all increase the risk of developing athlete's foot. In crowded living conditions where multiple people share bathrooms or washing areas, the fungi can easily spread from person to person.

Treatment for athlete's foot usually involves topical antifungal medications applied directly to the affected area. These medications need to be used consistently for several weeks, often continuing for a week or two after symptoms disappear to ensure the infection is completely eliminated.

Prevention of athlete's foot focuses on keeping feet clean and dry, wearing breathable footwear when possible, and avoiding walking barefoot in areas where fungal contamination is likely. In shared bathing facilities, wearing sandals or other protective footwear can help prevent infection.

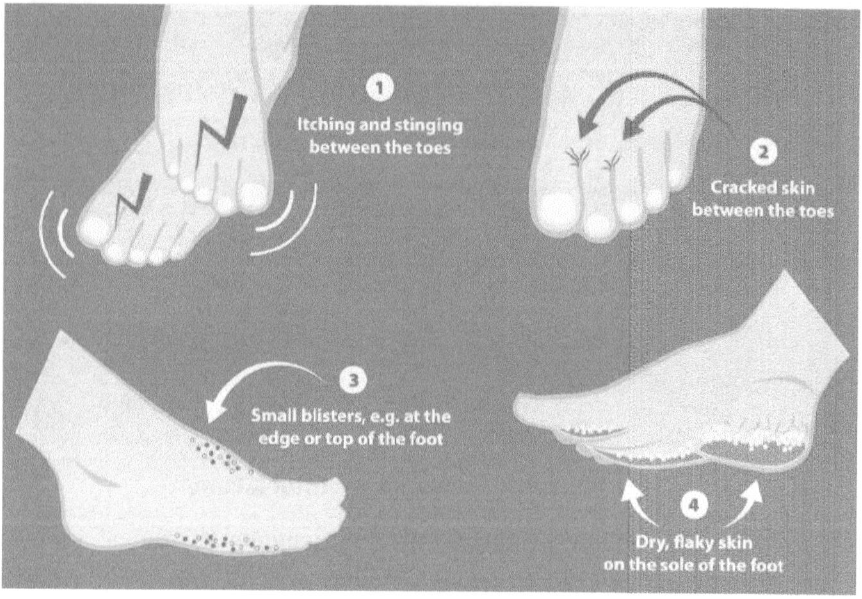

Pic 81: https://www.facebook.com/61571610214108/posts/%EF%B8%8F%EF%B8%8Flots-of-people-have-experienced- athletes-foot-and-are-aware-of-the-symptoms- of/122127703106720340/

Ringworm - The Circular Rash

Despite its name, ringworm is not caused by worms but by the same types of fungi that cause athlete's foot. The infection gets its name from the characteristic circular, ring-like rash it produces on the skin. Ringworm can affect any part of the body and is highly contagious.

Ringworm infections typically begin as small, red, scaly patches on the skin. As the infection spreads outward, the center of the patch often clears up, creating the characteristic ring appearance with a red, raised border and clearer skin in the center.

The infection can occur anywhere on the body but is most common on areas that are warm and moist or that come into frequent contact with contaminated surfaces.

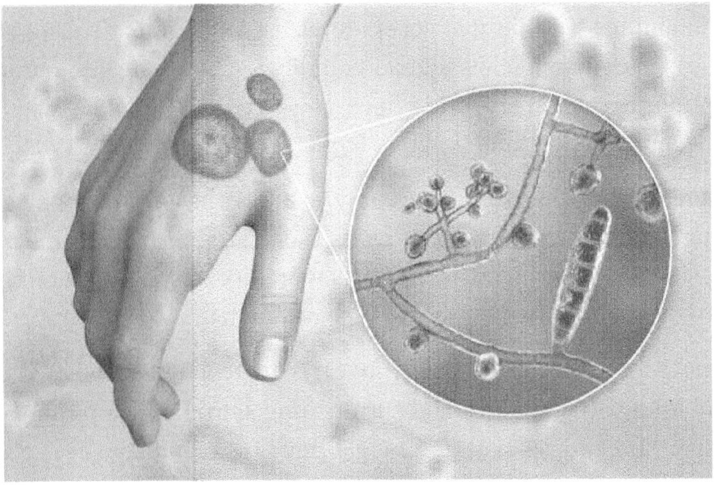

Pic 82: https://theconversation.com/

Common locations include the arms, legs, trunk, and scalp. Scalp ringworm is particularly common in children and can cause hair loss in the affected areas.

Ringworm spreads through direct contact with infected people or animals, or through contact with contaminated objects like clothing, towels, or surfaces. The fungi can survive on objects for extended periods, making transmission through shared items a significant concern in crowded living conditions.

Animals, particularly cats and dogs, can carry ringworm fungi and transmit them to humans. Farm animals and pets that are allowed to roam freely may become infected and then spread the infection to people who handle them.

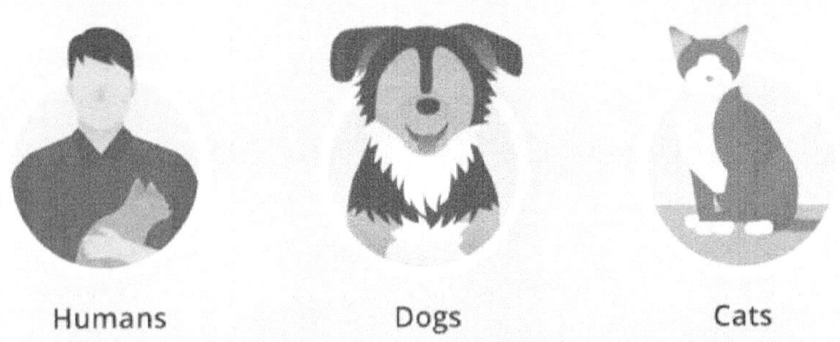

Pic 83: https://canna-pet.com/

In communities with limited access to clean water and adequate hygiene facilities, ringworm can spread rapidly. Children are particularly susceptible because they often have close physical contact with others and may not always maintain good hygiene practices.

The diagnosis of ringworm is usually made based on the appearance of the characteristic rash. In some cases, healthcare providers may take a small sample of affected skin for laboratory testing to confirm the diagnosis and identify the specific type of fungus.

Treatment for ringworm typically involves topical antifungal medications applied to the affected area and surrounding skin. For scalp ringworm or extensive infections, oral antifungal medications may be necessary. Treatment usually needs to continue for several weeks after the rash disappears.

Internal Fungal Infections

Thrush - In Mouth or Intimate Areas

Thrush is a fungal infection caused by an overgrowth of Candida yeasts, which normally live in small numbers in the mouth, digestive tract, and vaginal area without causing problems. When conditions allow these yeasts to multiply excessively, they can cause uncomfortable infections.

Oral thrush appears as white or cream-colored patches on the tongue, inside of the cheeks, or on the roof of the mouth. These patches may look like cottage cheese and can usually be wiped away, revealing red, irritated tissue underneath. The affected areas may be painful and can interfere with eating or drinking.

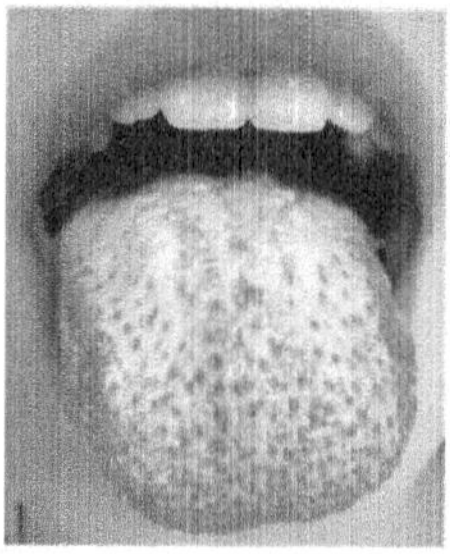

Pic 84: https://www.healthline.com/

Vaginal thrush, also called a yeast infection, causes itching, burning, and a thick, white discharge. The vulva may become red and swollen, and urination may be painful. Many women experience vaginal thrush at some point in their lives, and some have recurrent infections.

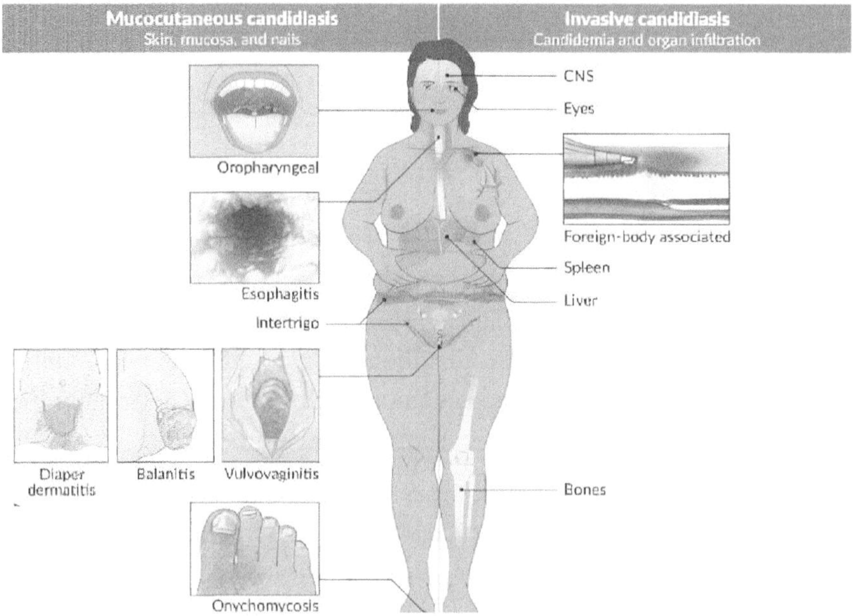

Pic 85: https://www.czvbz.store/?ggcid=485332

Several factors can increase the risk of developing thrush. Antibiotic use can disrupt the normal balance of bacteria and yeasts, allowing Candida to overgrow. Diabetes, particularly when blood sugar levels are poorly controlled, creates conditions that favor yeast growth.

Weakened immune systems, whether due to illness, stress, poor nutrition, or certain medications, can allow normally harmless yeasts to cause infections. Pregnancy, hormonal changes, and certain medical conditions can also increase susceptibility to thrush.

In crowded living conditions with limited access to clean water and hygiene facilities, thrush may be more common and more difficult to treat effectively. Poor nutrition can weaken immune defenses, making fungal infections more likely.

Treatment for thrush usually involves antifungal medications that can be applied topically or taken orally, depending on the location and severity of the infection. For oral thrush, antifungal mouth rinses or lozenges may be used. For vaginal thrush, antifungal creams or suppositories are typically prescribed.

Prevention of thrush involves maintaining good hygiene, avoiding unnecessary antibiotic use, managing underlying health conditions like diabetes, and supporting immune function through good nutrition and stress management.

When Fungi Become Serious

While most fungal infections are superficial and relatively minor, some can become serious, particularly in people with weakened immune systems or underlying health conditions. Understanding when fungal infections require urgent medical attention helps prevent potentially life-threatening complications.

Invasive fungal infections occur when fungi spread beyond the skin and superficial tissues to affect internal organs. These infections can affect the lungs, bloodstream, brain, or other vital organs and can be rapidly fatal if not promptly treated.

People with compromised immune systems are at highest risk for serious fungal infections. This includes people with HIV/AIDS, cancer patients receiving chemotherapy, organ transplant recipients taking immunosuppressive medications, and people with severe malnutrition.

Lung infections caused by fungi can resemble pneumonia and may be difficult to distinguish from bacterial or viral respiratory infections. Symptoms may include persistent cough, fever, chest pain, and difficulty breathing. Without proper treatment, fungal pneumonia can be fatal.

Bloodstream infections caused by fungi, called candidemia, are medical emergencies that require immediate treatment with intravenous antifungal medications. Symptoms may include fever, chills, and signs of sepsis such as low blood pressure and organ dysfunction.

Brain infections caused by fungi are rare but extremely serious. They can cause symptoms such as severe headache, confusion, seizures, and loss of consciousness. These infections require aggressive treatment and often result in permanent neurological damage even with appropriate care.

Chronic fungal infections can also cause serious health problems over time. For example, chronic lung infections can lead to progressive lung damage and respiratory failure. Chronic skin infections can become extensively disfiguring and may predispose to bacterial infections.

Vector-Borne Diseases

Mosquito-Transmitted Diseases

Malaria - Prevention and Recognition

Prevention of malaria focuses primarily on reducing exposure to infected mosquitoes, since there is no vaccine available for most strains of malaria parasites. Understanding mosquito behavior and breeding patterns helps communities develop effective prevention strategies.

Anopheles mosquitoes, which transmit malaria, are most active during twilight and nighttime hours. They prefer to bite people indoors during the evening and night, making protection during sleep particularly important. These mosquitoes are also attracted to dark colors and carbon dioxide from human breath.

Insecticide-treated bed nets are one of the most effective tools for preventing malaria. These nets create a physical barrier between sleeping people and mosquitoes, and the insecticide kills mosquitoes that come into contact with the net. For maximum effectiveness, nets should completely cover the sleeping area and be tucked under mattresses or sleeping mats.

Proper use and maintenance of bed nets is crucial for their effectiveness. Nets should be checked regularly for holes and repaired promptly. They should be retreated with insecticide according to manufacturer recommendations, typically every six months to two years depending on the type of net.

Indoor residual spraying involves applying long-lasting insecticides to the walls and ceilings of homes. When mosquitoes rest on these treated surfaces after feeding, they absorb lethal doses of insecticide. This method can provide protection for entire communities when implemented systematically.

Environmental management to reduce mosquito breeding sites is another important prevention strategy. This includes eliminating standing water around homes, improving drainage to prevent water accumulation, and managing water storage to minimize mosquito breeding opportunities.

Personal protective measures can provide additional protection, particularly for people who must be active during peak mosquito hours. These include wearing long-sleeved clothing and long pants, using insect repellents containing DEET or other effective ingredients, and avoiding outdoor activities during dusk and dawn when mosquitoes are most active.

Dengue Fever - The Urban Threat

Dengue fever is a viral infection transmitted by Aedes aegypti mosquitoes, which have different behavior patterns than the Anopheles mosquitoes that transmit malaria. Understanding these differences is important for developing appropriate prevention strategies.

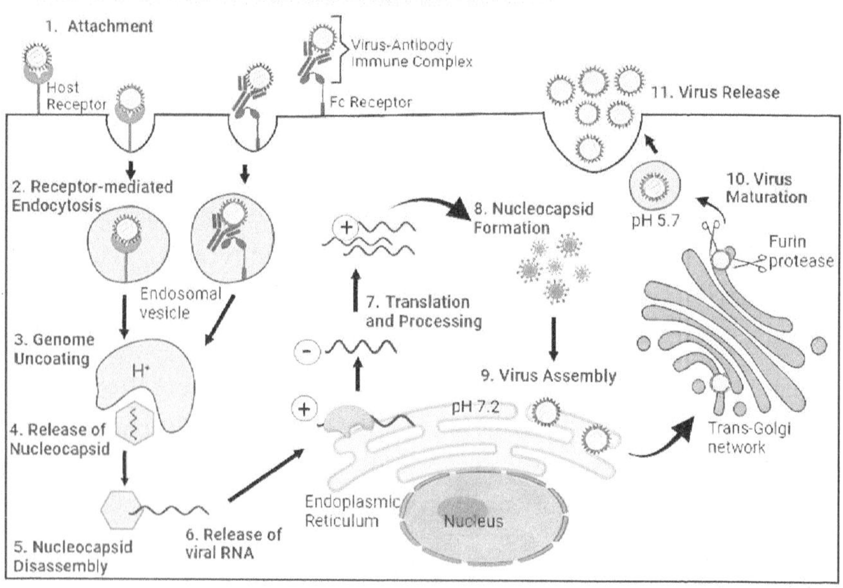

Pic 86: https://jbiomedsci.biomedcentral.com/

Unlike malaria mosquitoes, Aedes aegypti mosquitoes are active during daylight hours, particularly during early morning and late afternoon. They prefer to bite people outdoors and are commonly found in urban and semi-urban areas where they breed in artificial water containers.

Dengue has become increasingly common in crowded urban areas where Aedes mosquitoes thrive. These mosquitoes breed in clean, standing water found in containers like storage tanks, flower pots, discarded tires, and any other objects that can collect rainwater.

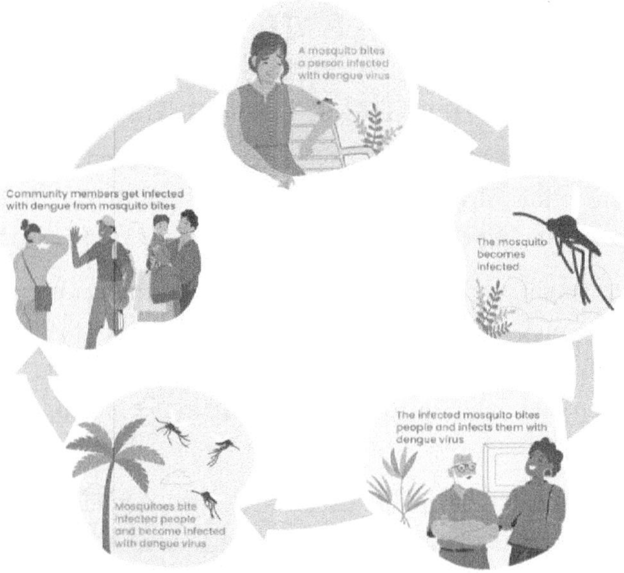

Pic 87: https://www.cdc.gov/dengue/transmission/index.html

The symptoms of dengue fever typically begin 4-7 days after being bitten by an infected mosquito. Early symptoms include sudden onset of high fever, severe headache, pain behind the eyes, muscle and joint pains, and skin rash. These symptoms can be mistaken for other illnesses, making diagnosis challenging.

Severe dengue, also known as dengue hemorrhagic fever, can develop as the fever begins to subside, typically 3-5 days after symptom onset. Warning signs include severe abdominal pain, persistent vomiting, rapid breathing, bleeding gums, blood in vomit, and extreme restlessness. Severe dengue can be fatal without proper medical care.

There is no specific treatment for dengue fever, so management focuses on maintaining proper fluid balance and monitoring for complications. Aspirin should be avoided because it can increase bleeding risk. Paracetamol can be used for fever control, but patients should be monitored carefully for signs of severe dengue.

Prevention of dengue focuses on eliminating mosquito breeding sites around homes and communities. This requires community- wide efforts to remove or properly manage water storage containers, clean up areas where water can accumulate, and educate residents about mosquito control.

Other Vectors - Flies, Ticks, Contaminated Water

Many other insects and contaminated water sources can transmit parasitic and other infectious diseases. Understanding these diverse transmission routes helps communities develop comprehensive prevention strategies.

Flies can transmit various diseases through mechanical transmission, meaning they pick up pathogens on their bodies and transfer them to food or surfaces. House flies can carry bacteria that cause diarrheal diseases when they land on food after contacting contaminated waste or garbage.

Tsetse flies transmit sleeping sickness (trypanosomiasis) in parts of Africa. These flies are active during daylight hours and are attracted to moving objects, bright colors, and dark blue clothing. Prevention involves avoiding areas where tsetse flies are common and wearing appropriate protective clothing.

Ticks can transmit various diseases including Rocky Mountain spotted fever, Lyme disease, and tick-borne relapsing fever. Ticks attach to people or animals walking through grass or wooded areas where ticks are present. Prevention includes wearing protective clothing, using insect repellents, and checking for ticks after spending time in potentially infested areas.

Contaminated water can transmit many parasitic diseases including giardiasis, cryptosporidiosis, and various worm infections. These parasites can survive in water for extended periods and are often resistant to standard water treatment methods.

Sand flies transmit leishmaniasis, a parasitic disease that can affect the skin or internal organs. These tiny flies are most active during warm, humid evenings and are found in many tropical and subtropical areas. Prevention involves using bed nets, wearing protective clothing, and avoiding outdoor activities during peak sand fly hours.

Black flies transmit river blindness (onchocerciasis) in parts of Africa and Latin America. These flies breed in fast-flowing rivers and streams and bite during daylight hours. Prevention involves avoiding areas near breeding sites and using protective clothing and repellents.

Community Focus: Sanitation and Vector Control

Water Management - Reducing Mosquito Breeding

Effective mosquito control requires community-wide water management strategies that address both natural and artificial breeding sites. These efforts are most successful when entire communities participate and when they are sustained over time.

Artificial water containers provide ideal breeding sites for many disease-carrying mosquitoes. In urban and semi-urban areas, these containers may include water storage tanks, buckets, flower pots, discarded tires, plastic containers, and any other objects that can collect and hold water.

Proper water storage is essential for preventing mosquito breeding while maintaining access to clean water for household use. Water storage containers should be covered with tight-fitting lids or screens that prevent mosquitoes from entering. Containers should be cleaned regularly to remove any eggs or larvae that may be present.

Large water storage tanks should be inspected regularly for cracks or openings that could allow mosquito entry. Even small openings can provide access for female mosquitoes seeking places to lay eggs. Covers should be secure and should not allow water to accumulate on top.

Drainage improvements can significantly reduce mosquito breeding opportunities. Poor drainage around homes and communities creates puddles and standing water where mosquitoes can breed. Simple drainage ditches, proper grading of land around homes, and maintenance of existing drainage systems can eliminate many breeding sites.

Rainwater harvesting systems, while beneficial for water security, can create mosquito breeding sites if not properly designed and maintained. These systems should include screens, covers, and regular maintenance to prevent mosquito access while preserving water quality.

Community water sources like wells, springs, and ponds may also serve as mosquito breeding sites. While these sources are important for community water supply, they may need modification to reduce mosquito breeding without compromising water access.

Waste Management - Breaking Parasite Cycles

Proper waste management is crucial for preventing the transmission of many parasitic diseases. Human waste, in particular, can contaminate water and soil with parasite eggs and larvae, creating ongoing cycles of infection and reinfection.

Adequate toilet facilities that safely contain human waste are essential for breaking transmission cycles of intestinal worms and other parasites. Toilets should be located away from water sources and should be designed to prevent contamination of groundwater.

In areas where flush toilets are not feasible, pit latrines or composting toilets can provide safe waste disposal if properly constructed and maintained. These facilities should be covered to prevent flies from accessing waste and should be located downhill from water sources.

Solid waste management also plays a role in disease prevention. Garbage and organic waste can attract flies and rodents that can transmit diseases. Regular waste collection or proper disposal methods help reduce these disease vectors.

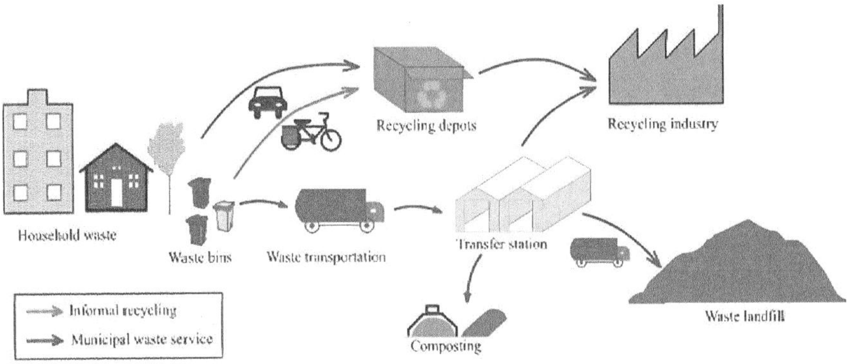

Pic 88: https://www.researchgate.net/figure/The-waste-management-cycle_fig1_311161719

Food waste should be disposed of promptly and properly to avoid attracting flies and other pests. Composting can be an effective way to manage organic waste while creating useful soil amendments, but compost piles should be properly managed to prevent them from becoming breeding sites for disease vectors.

Animal waste from livestock or pets should also be managed properly. Animal feces can contain parasites that can infect humans, so these wastes should be disposed of away from areas where people live, work, or play.

Community Education - Recognizing and Reporting Cases

Education about parasite and vector-borne diseases helps communities recognize cases early, seek appropriate treatment, and implement prevention measures. Effective education programs use culturally appropriate methods and involve community leaders and trusted figures.

Teaching community members to recognize the symptoms of common parasitic diseases helps ensure that cases are identified and treated promptly. Early treatment often prevents complications and reduces the risk of transmission to others.

Education about transmission routes helps people understand how they can protect themselves and their families. This includes information about mosquito breeding sites, safe water practices, proper hygiene, and food safety.

Community health workers can play crucial roles in education and case detection. These workers, who are often community members themselves, can provide ongoing education, help identify cases, and connect people with appropriate treatment resources.

Reporting systems help health authorities track disease patterns and respond to outbreaks. Community members should know how to report cases of serious diseases like malaria, dengue, or unusual clusters of illness.

Schools provide important opportunities for education about disease prevention. Children can learn prevention practices that they can share with their families, and they can be monitored for signs of common childhood parasitic infections.

Low-Cost Prevention - Bed Nets, Proper Toilets, Clean Water

Effective prevention of parasitic and vector-borne diseases doesn't always require expensive interventions. Many low-cost strategies can significantly reduce disease transmission when implemented consistently across communities.

Bed nets, particularly insecticide-treated nets, provide excellent protection against malaria and other mosquito-borne diseases at relatively low cost. Community programs that distribute nets and provide education about proper use can dramatically reduce disease transmission.

Simple improvements to water storage and handling can prevent many waterborne parasitic infections. Using covered containers, treating water when necessary, and practicing good hygiene around water sources are low-cost interventions with significant health benefits.

Basic sanitation improvements, including simple pit latrines or composting toilets, can break transmission cycles for many parasitic diseases. While initial construction requires some investment, these facilities can serve families for many years with proper maintenance.

Community clean-up efforts that eliminate mosquito breeding sites cost little beyond community time and effort but can significantly reduce vector populations. Regular community days focused on removing standing water and cleaning up breeding sites can be highly effective.

Personal protective measures like wearing long sleeves and pants during peak mosquito hours, using locally available repellents, and avoiding known breeding areas can provide significant protection at minimal cost.

Chapter - 8
Medicines That Help - Using Treatments Safely

"The right medicine for the right problem"

Understanding Different Medicine Types

Antibiotics - For Bacterial Infections Only

Antibiotics represent one of the greatest medical advances in human history, transforming bacterial infections from frequently fatal diseases to manageable conditions. However, understanding how antibiotics work and when they should be used is crucial for maintaining their effectiveness and avoiding harm.

Antibiotics are specifically designed to kill bacteria or prevent them from reproducing. They work by targeting specific features of bacterial cells that are different from human cells, allowing them to eliminate bacteria while causing minimal harm to the human body. This specificity is both the strength and limitation of antibiotic therapy.

Different classes of antibiotics work through different mechanisms. Penicillins and related antibiotics attack the bacterial cell wall, causing bacteria to burst and die. These antibiotics are particularly effective against bacteria that have thick cell walls, though some bacteria have developed resistance by producing enzymes that break down penicillin.

Tetracyclines and similar antibiotics interfere with bacterial protein synthesis by binding to bacterial ribosomes. Since bacteria need to make proteins to survive and reproduce, blocking protein synthesis effectively kills or stops bacterial growth. These antibiotics are effective against a wide range of bacteria.

Fluoroquinolones work by interfering with bacterial DNA replication and repair. They block enzymes that bacteria need to copy their genetic material, preventing bacterial reproduction. These antibiotics are often used for serious infections that don't respond to other treatments.

The key principle in antibiotic use is that these medicines only work against bacterial infections. They have no effect whatsoever on viral infections, fungal infections, or parasitic infections. Using antibiotics for non-bacterial infections is not only ineffective but can cause harm by disrupting beneficial bacteria and contributing to antibiotic resistance.

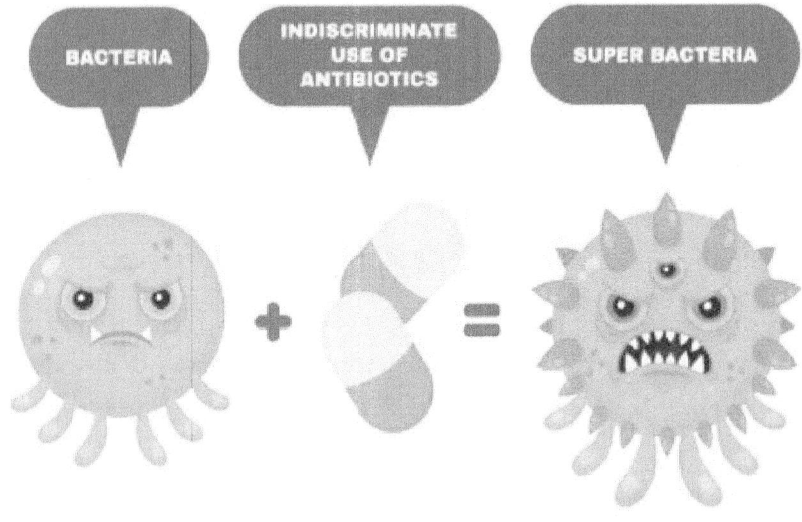

Pic 89: https://www.dreamstime.com/

Misuse of antibiotics, such as taking them without prescription, not completing the full course, or using them for viral infections, allows harmful bacteria to survive and adapt. Over time, these surviving bacteria become resistant, leading to the rise of dangerous drug-resistant "superbugs" that are difficult to treat.

Proper antibiotic use requires taking the complete prescribed course, even when symptoms improve before the medicine is finished. This ensures that all bacteria are eliminated and reduces the chance that resistant bacteria will survive and multiply.

Antivirals - Rare but Important for Some Viruses

Antiviral medications are much less common than antibiotics and are available for only a limited number of viral infections. Unlike antibiotics, which can treat many different bacterial infections, most antiviral drugs are designed to work against specific viruses.

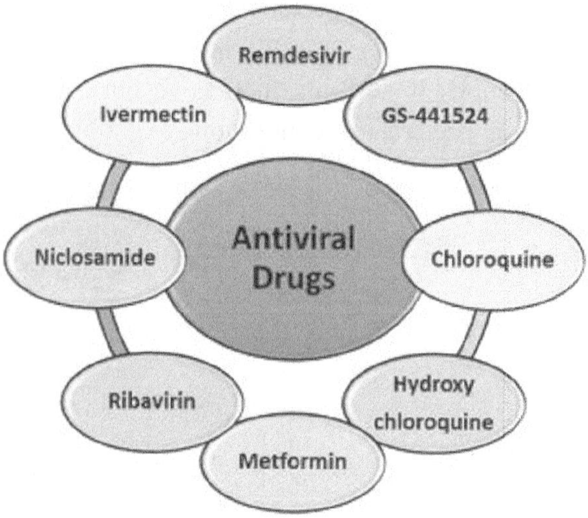

Pic 90: https://www.researchgate.net/figure/Antiviral- drugs-against-COVID-19_fig3_358682492

The development of antiviral drugs is challenging because viruses live inside human cells and use the host cell's machinery to reproduce. Any drug that interferes with viral reproduction must be able to distinguish between viral processes and normal human cellular processes, which is technically difficult.

Most antiviral drugs work by interfering with specific steps in viral reproduction. Some block the virus from entering cells, others prevent the virus from making copies of its genetic material, and still others interfere with the assembly of new viral particles.

Oseltamivir (Tamiflu) is one of the most commonly used antiviral drugs and is designed specifically to treat influenza infections. It works by blocking an enzyme that influenza viruses need to spread from infected cells to healthy cells. When used within 48 hours of symptom onset, it can reduce the duration and severity of flu symptoms.

Acyclovir and related drugs are used to treat infections caused by herpes viruses, including oral herpes, genital herpes, and chickenpox. These drugs work by interfering with viral DNA replication, preventing the virus from making copies of itself.

Antiretroviral drugs used to treat HIV infection represent one of the most successful examples of antiviral therapy. These drugs work by blocking different steps in the HIV life cycle, and when used in combination, they can suppress viral replication to undetectable levels.

For most viral infections, including the common cold, flu (when antiviral treatment is not available or appropriate), and many childhood viral infections, supportive care remains the primary treatment approach. This includes rest, adequate fluid intake, fever management, and monitoring for complications.

Anti-Parasitics - For Worms and Other Parasites

Anti-parasitic medications are designed to eliminate various types of parasites that can infect humans. These drugs work through different mechanisms depending on the type of parasite they target, and proper selection of anti-parasitic treatment requires understanding what type of parasite is causing the infection.

Anthelmintics are medications specifically designed to treat worm infections. Different anthelmintics work through different mechanisms, and some are effective against multiple types of worms while others are specific to particular species.

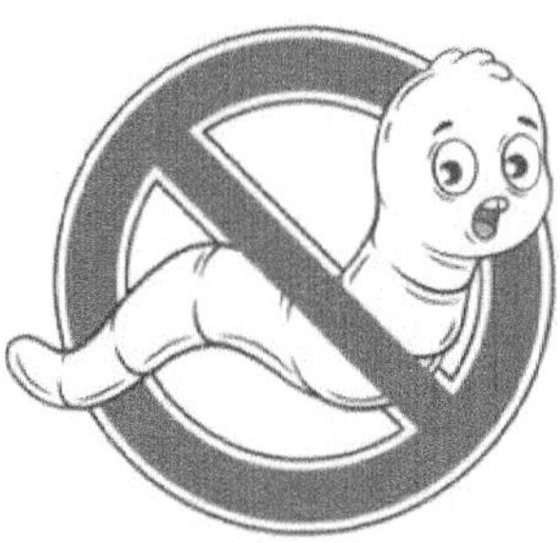

Pic 91: https://www.dreamstime.com/stop-worm- helminth-parasite-plant-pest-insect-control-icon-anthelmintic-medicine-insecticide-garden-parasitic-larva- bug-image238542159

Mebendazole and albendazole are broad-spectrum anthelmintics that work by interfering with the worms' ability to absorb nutrients. These medications are effective against many common intestinal worms including roundworms, hookworms, and whipworms. They are often used in mass treatment programs because of their broad effectiveness and safety profile.

Praziquantel is particularly effective against tapeworms and schistosomiasis. It works by causing paralysis in the parasites, allowing the body's immune system to eliminate them. This medication requires careful dosing based on body weight and the specific type of parasite being treated.

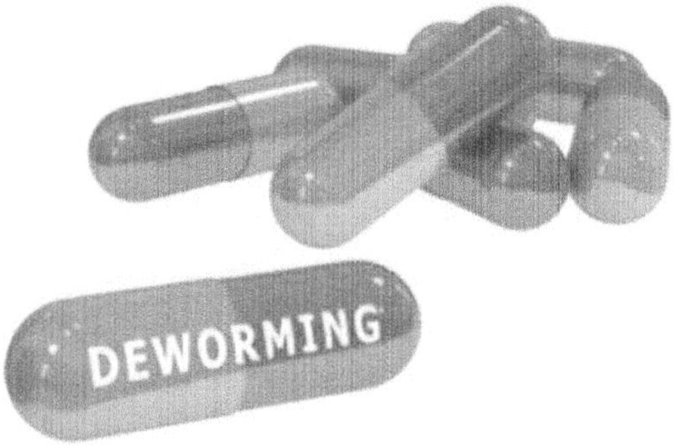

Pic 92: https://www.shutterstock.com/

Antimalarial drugs work by interfering with the malaria parasite's life cycle inside human red blood cells. Different antimalarials work through different mechanisms, and the choice of medication depends on the species of malaria parasite and local patterns of drug resistance.

Chloroquine was once widely used for malaria treatment but is now ineffective in many areas due to resistance. Artemisinin-based combination therapies (ACTs) are now the recommended first-line treatment for uncomplicated malaria in most areas where resistance to chloroquine has developed.

For other parasitic infections, specific medications may be required. Metronidazole is commonly used for parasitic infections of the digestive system like giardiasis and amoebiasis. Ivermectin is effective against certain parasitic worm infections and external parasites like scabies.

Antifungals - For Fungal Infections

Antifungal medications treat infections caused by fungi, including yeasts like Candida and molds like those that cause ringworm and athlete's foot. Like other antimicrobial drugs, antifungals work by targeting features of fungal cells that are different from human cells.

Topical antifungals are applied directly to infected skin, nails, or mucous membranes. These medications include creams, ointments, powders, and solutions that can be applied to affected areas. Common topical antifungals include clotrimazole, miconazole, and terbinafine.

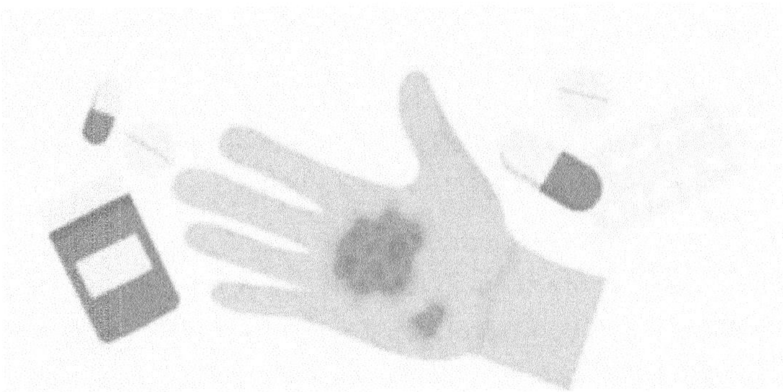

Pic 93: https://www.vecteezy.com/

For superficial fungal infections like athlete's foot, ringworm, and yeast infections, topical treatments are usually sufficient. These medications need to be applied consistently for the full recommended duration, often continuing for a week or two after symptoms disappear to ensure complete elimination of the fungus.

Oral antifungal medications are used for more extensive infections, infections that don't respond to topical treatment, or infections in areas where topical application is difficult. These medications can have more side effects than topical treatments and may interact with other medications.

Fluconazole is commonly used for yeast infections and can be taken orally for vaginal yeast infections or thrush. It's generally well-tolerated but can interact with other medications and should be used carefully in people with liver problems.

For serious, invasive fungal infections that affect internal organs, more potent antifungal medications may be required. These infections are relatively rare but can be life-threatening, particularly in people with compromised immune systems.

The Danger of Wrong Medicine Use

Self-Medication Risks - Why Guessing Can Be Dangerous

Self-medication, while sometimes necessary in areas with limited access to healthcare, carries significant risks that can lead to treatment failure, drug resistance, and serious adverse effects.

Understanding these risks helps people make safer decisions about when to self-treat and when to seek professional help.

Using the wrong type of medication for an infection can delay proper treatment and allow infections to worsen. For example, taking antibiotics for viral infections not only provides no benefit but may mask symptoms that could help healthcare providers make correct diagnoses later.

Incorrect dosing is a common problem with self-medication. Taking too little medication may not eliminate the infection completely, allowing resistant organisms to survive and multiply. Taking too much medication increases the risk of side effects and toxicity without providing additional benefits.

Many medications can interact with other drugs, foods, or underlying health conditions in ways that can be dangerous. People who self-medicate may not be aware of these interactions, particularly if they're taking multiple medications or have health conditions they don't fully understand.

Some infections require specific diagnostic tests to identify the exact cause and guide appropriate treatment. Self-medication based on symptoms alone may target the wrong organism or miss serious complications that require different treatment approaches.

Allergic reactions to medications can be severe and life- threatening. People who self-medicate may not be aware of allergies to specific medications, and they may not recognize the early signs of allergic reactions that require immediate medical attention.

Self-medication can also mask symptoms of serious underlying conditions. For example, taking pain relievers for abdominal pain might temporarily reduce discomfort but could delay diagnosis of conditions like appendicitis that require emergency treatment.

Counterfeit Drugs in Slums - How to Spot Fake Medicines

Counterfeit medications are a serious problem in many communities with limited healthcare resources. These fake medicines can contain wrong ingredients, no active ingredients, or harmful substances, making them ineffective or dangerous.

Counterfeit drugs often have subtle differences in packaging, labeling, or appearance compared to genuine medications. However, these differences can be difficult to detect without careful examination and knowledge of what to look for.

Unusually low prices can be a warning sign of counterfeit medications. While price alone is not a reliable indicator, medicines sold at prices significantly below normal market rates should be viewed with suspicion, especially if they're being sold in unofficial locations.

The source of medications is important for ensuring authenticity. Medicines purchased from licensed pharmacies, healthcare facilities, or authorized distributors are much more likely to be genuine than those purchased from street vendors, unmarked shops, or door-to-door sellers.

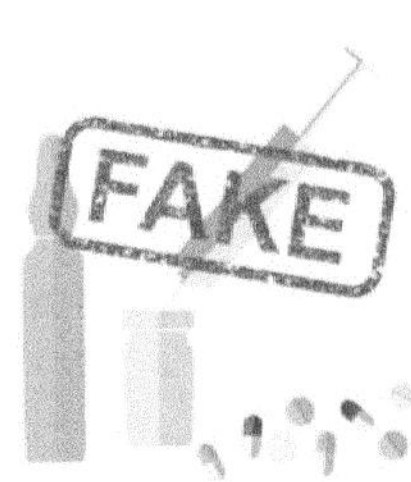

Pic 94: https://www.shutterstock.com/

Packaging quality can provide clues about medication authenticity. Genuine medications typically have high-quality packaging with clear, professional printing and proper sealing. Poor-quality packaging, unclear printing, or damaged seals may indicate counterfeit products.

Expiration dates and batch numbers should be clearly marked on all genuine medications. Packages without this information, or with dates that appear to have been altered or overprinted, should be considered suspicious.

Some countries have systems for verifying medication authenticity, such as QR codes or text message verification systems. When available, these systems can help confirm that medications are genuine.

Incomplete Treatments - Why Stopping Early Causes Problems

One of the most dangerous practices in medication use is stopping treatment early when symptoms improve but the full course of medicine hasn't been completed. This practice can lead to treatment failure, relapse of infection, and development of drug resistance.

For bacterial infections, incomplete antibiotic treatment allows some bacteria to survive, often those that are most resistant to the antibiotic being used. These surviving bacteria can multiply and cause the infection to return, but now the same antibiotic may be less effective or completely ineffective.

The bacteria that survive incomplete treatment can also spread to other people, potentially causing infections that are more difficult to treat from the beginning. This contributes to the community- wide problem of antibiotic resistance.

For parasitic infections, incomplete treatment can also lead to treatment failure and resistance. Many anti-parasitic medications work slowly, and it may take several days or weeks to eliminate all parasites from the body. Stopping treatment early allows parasites to recover and continue causing infection.

The symptoms of infections often improve before all the disease- causing organisms have been eliminated from the body. This is because the medication reduces the number of organisms to levels that the immune system can control, reducing symptoms even though some organisms remain.

Completing the full course of treatment ensures that medication levels in the body remain high enough for long enough to eliminate all disease-causing organisms. This reduces the chance of relapse and prevents the development of resistance.

For chronic conditions like tuberculosis, incomplete treatment is particularly dangerous because it can lead to drug-resistant forms of the disease that are much more difficult and expensive to treat.

Sharing Medicines - Why Your Medicine Might Hurt Others

Sharing prescription medications between family members or friends is a common practice in many communities, particularly when healthcare access is limited or expensive. However, this practice can be dangerous for several important reasons.

Different people may need different types or amounts of medication, even for infections that appear similar. What works for one person may not work for another due to differences in the type of organism causing infection, the severity of infection, or individual factors like body weight and kidney function.

Shared medications may not provide enough treatment to cure an infection completely. When people share a prescribed course of medication, each person typically receives less than the full recommended dose, increasing the risk of treatment failure and resistance development.

Some people may have allergies or medical conditions that make certain medications dangerous for them. Without proper medical evaluation, shared medications could cause serious adverse reactions in people who shouldn't take those particular drugs.

Medications that are safe and appropriate for adults may be dangerous for children, or may require different dosing based on age and weight. Sharing adult medications with children can lead to overdosing or other serious complications.

Some medications can interact with other drugs that people may be taking. These interactions can reduce effectiveness or cause dangerous side effects. Healthcare providers consider these potential interactions when prescribing medications, but people sharing medications may not be aware of these risks.

The person sharing their medication may not complete their own full course of treatment, which can lead to treatment failure and relapse of their own infection.

Community Focus: Safe Medicine Practices Trusted Sources - Where to Get Real Medicines

Identifying reliable sources of genuine medications is crucial for ensuring both safety and effectiveness of treatment. In communities with limited healthcare infrastructure, this can be challenging but remains essential for good health outcomes.

Licensed pharmacies are generally the most reliable sources of genuine medications. These establishments are required to meet certain standards for storage, handling, and dispensing of medications. They typically have trained staff who can provide basic information about proper medication use.

Healthcare facilities including hospitals, clinics, and health centers usually maintain reliable supplies of essential medications. While the selection may be limited, medications obtained from these sources are more likely to be genuine and properly stored.

Government health programs often provide medications for common conditions like malaria, tuberculosis, and childhood diseases. These programs typically have quality control measures in place to ensure medication authenticity and effectiveness.

Pradhan Mantri Bhartiya Janaushadhi Kendras (PMBJKs) are government-run pharmacies that provide quality generic medicines at affordable prices to the public. These medicines are as effective as branded ones but cost much less, making healthcare accessible to all. The initiative helps reduce out-of-pocket medical expenses, especially for poor and middle-class families. It also spreads awareness about the benefits of using generic medicines over costly branded alternatives.

Non-governmental organizations (NGOs) and international aid organizations may also provide reliable sources of medications in some areas. These organizations usually have quality control procedures and work with reputable suppliers.

Community health workers who are properly trained and supplied through official health programs can be reliable sources of certain medications, particularly for common conditions like malaria, diarrhea, and respiratory infections.

Avoiding unreliable sources is equally important for medication safety. Street vendors, door-to-door sellers, and informal markets are more likely to sell counterfeit or expired medications.

Medicines sold at extremely low prices or in unusual locations should be viewed with suspicion.

Following Instructions - Dose, Timing, Duration

Proper medication use requires careful attention to dosing instructions, timing of doses, and duration of treatment. These factors are designed to ensure maximum effectiveness while minimizing the risk of side effects and resistance development.

Dosing instructions specify how much medication to take and are usually based on factors like body weight, age, severity of infection, and kidney function. Taking too little medication may not eliminate the infection completely, while taking too much increases the risk of side effects without providing additional benefits.

The timing of doses is important for maintaining effective levels of medication in the body. Some medications need to be taken at regular intervals throughout the day to maintain constant levels in the bloodstream. Others may be designed for once-daily dosing.

Taking medications with or without food can affect how well they're absorbed and how they work in the body. Some medications should be taken on an empty stomach for best absorption, while others should be taken with food to reduce stomach irritation.

The total duration of treatment is designed to ensure complete elimination of the infection. This duration is based on research showing how long it takes for specific medications to eliminate particular types of infections. Stopping treatment early, even when symptoms improve, can lead to treatment failure.

Some medications require special timing considerations. For example, antimalarial medications may need to be started before travel to malaria-endemic areas and continued for a period after leaving these areas.

Storage and Expiration - Keeping Medicines Effective

Proper storage of medications is essential for maintaining their effectiveness and safety. Many medications can lose potency or become dangerous if not stored correctly, particularly in hot, humid climates.

Temperature control is crucial for many medications. Most medicines should be stored at room temperature, away from heat sources like stoves, direct sunlight, or hot vehicles. Some medications require refrigeration, though this can be challenging in areas without reliable electricity.

Humidity can also affect medication stability. Many medications should be kept in dry places and protected from moisture. Bathroom storage is often not ideal because of humidity from showers and baths.

Original packaging helps protect medications from light, moisture, and contamination. Medications should generally be kept in their original containers with original labels until they're used completely.

Expiration dates indicate how long medications remain effective and safe when stored properly. Using expired medications may be ineffective and, in some cases, dangerous. Expired medications should be disposed of properly rather than being saved for future use.

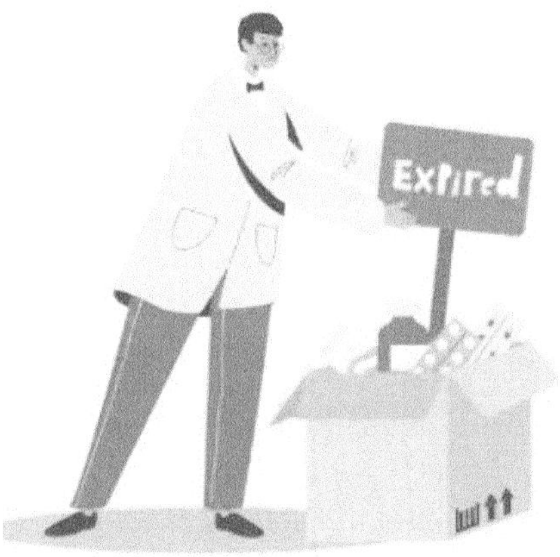

Pic 95: https://www.freepik.com/

Some medications have special storage requirements. Liquid medications may need refrigeration and should be shaken before use if indicated. Eye drops and other sterile preparations have limited shelf lives once opened and should be discarded after the recommended period.

In hot climates, special attention should be paid to protecting medications from excessive heat. This might include using insulated containers for transport and avoiding storage in vehicles or other areas that become very hot.

When to Seek Medical Help - Don't Delay for Serious Infections

While some infections can be safely managed at home with appropriate medications, recognizing when professional medical care is needed can be life-saving. Certain warning signs indicate that infections are serious or that complications may be developing.

High fever, particularly in young children or elderly adults, often indicates serious infection that requires professional evaluation. Fever above 103°F (39.4°C) in adults or any fever in infants under three months old requires immediate medical attention.

Signs of severe dehydration include excessive thirst, dry mouth, little or no urination, dizziness when standing, and confusion. Severe dehydration can be life-threatening and may require intravenous fluid replacement.

Difficulty breathing, chest pain, or rapid breathing can indicate serious respiratory infections like pneumonia. These symptoms require prompt medical evaluation and may require antibiotic treatment or hospitalization.

Severe abdominal pain, particularly if it worsens over time, can indicate serious infections or other conditions that require immediate medical attention. Appendicitis, gallbladder infections, and other serious conditions can be life-threatening without prompt treatment.

Signs of bloodstream infection (sepsis) include high fever or low body temperature, rapid heart rate, rapid breathing, confusion, and signs of organ dysfunction. Sepsis is a medical emergency that requires immediate hospitalization and intensive treatment.

Infections that don't improve with appropriate treatment after 48-

72 hours may require different medications or professional evaluation to rule out complications or resistant organisms.

Any infection in someone with a compromised immune system, diabetes, heart disease, or other serious underlying conditions should be evaluated by healthcare providers because these conditions increase the risk of complications.

People should also seek medical care when they're unsure about the type of infection they have or what treatment is appropriate. Professional diagnosis can ensure that the right treatment is used from the beginning, improving outcomes and reducing the risk of complications.

Part III: Protecting Our Families

Keeping Our Loved Ones Healthy and Safe

Chapter - 9
Children's Health and Vaccinations

"Protecting our most vulnerable"

Why Children Get Sick More Often Developing Immune Systems

Children get sick more often than adults because their immune systems are still learning. Think of a child's immune system like a new security guard who hasn't seen many troublemakers yet. Each time the immune system fights off a new germ, it learns to recognize that germ and can fight it better next time.

Babies are born with some protection from their mothers, but this protection fades during their first year of life. This is why babies need extra care and protection from infections during their early months.

As children grow and encounter more germs, their immune systems become stronger and better at fighting infections. By the time they become adults, their immune systems have learned to recognize and fight many different types of germs.

Close Contact with Other Children

Children often play closely together, sharing toys, touching each other, and putting things in their mouths. This natural behavior helps them learn and develop, but it also makes it easy for germs to spread from child to child.

In schools, daycare centers, or when children play together in groups, one sick child can quickly spread illness to many others. Children may not understand or remember to cover their coughs, wash their hands, or avoid sharing food and drinks.

Less Developed Hygiene Habits

Young children are still learning good hygiene habits. They may forget to wash their hands, touch dirty surfaces and then touch their faces, or put contaminated objects in their mouths.

Children also breathe faster than adults, which means they take in more air and any germs floating in it. Their airways are smaller, so even minor swelling from infections can cause more serious breathing problems than in adults.

Physical Development Factors

Children's bodies are still growing and developing. Their airways, digestive systems, and other organs are smaller and may not work as efficiently as adult organs when fighting infections.

Because children are smaller, the same number of germs can cause more serious illness in a child than in an adult. They can also become dehydrated more quickly during illnesses that cause vomiting or diarrhea.

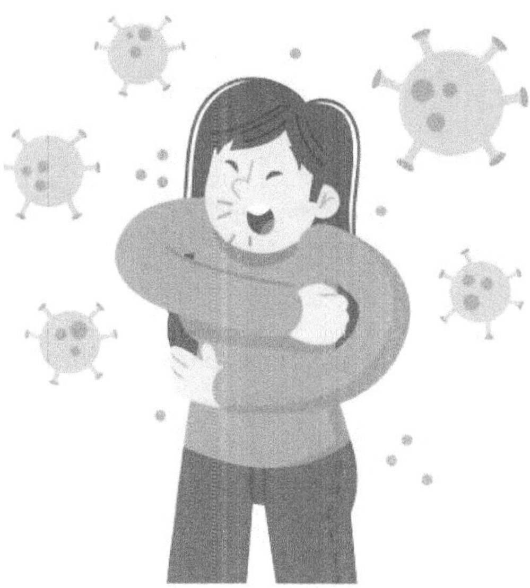

Pic 96: https://www.freepik.com/

How Vaccines Train the Immune System What Vaccines Are

Vaccines are like practice sessions for your immune system. They contain weakened or dead germs, or parts of germs, that cannot make you sick but can teach your immune system what these germs look like.

When you get a vaccine, your immune system learns to recognize the germ and creates memory cells that remember how to fight it. If the real germ ever tries to infect you, your immune system can quickly make antibodies to destroy it before you get sick.

How Vaccination Works

Getting vaccinated is like showing your immune system a wanted poster of a criminal. Your immune system studies the poster (the vaccine) and learns to recognize the criminal (the disease-causing germ).

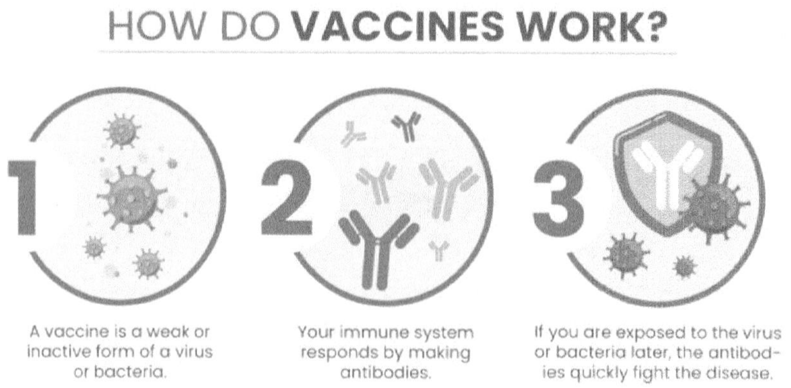

Pic 97: https://www.parsemus.org/

If that criminal ever shows up in your neighborhood (your body), your immune system security guards immediately recognize the threat and can arrest it (fight the infection) before it can cause trouble (make you sick).

Some vaccines need to be given multiple times to help your immune system remember the germ really well. This is called a series of shots. Booster shots later in life help refresh your immune system's memory.

Types of Vaccine Protection

Some vaccines give you direct protection - they prevent you from getting the disease at all. Others may not completely prevent infection but make the illness much milder if you do get sick.

Vaccines also provide community protection. When most people in a community are vaccinated against a disease, it becomes very hard for that disease to spread. This protects people who cannot be vaccinated due to illness or age.

This community protection is especially important for protecting babies who are too young to be vaccinated and people with weak immune systems who may not respond well to vaccines.

Essential Vaccines and When to Get Them

Vaccines for Babies and Young Children

BCG vaccine (for tuberculosis): Usually given at birth or within the first few months of life. This vaccine helps protect against severe forms of tuberculosis, which can be very dangerous in young children.

Hepatitis B vaccine: Usually given as a series starting at birth. This vaccine protects against a liver infection that can cause lifelong health problems.

DPT vaccine (Diphtheria, Pertussis, Tetanus): Given as a series starting at 6-8 weeks of age. This combination vaccine protects against three serious diseases:

- Diphtheria can cause breathing problems and heart damage
- Pertussis (whooping cough) causes severe coughing that can be life-threatening in babies
- Tetanus causes severe muscle spasms and can be fatal

Polio vaccine: Given as a series to prevent polio, which can cause permanent paralysis. Thanks to vaccination, polio has been eliminated from most of the world.

MMR vaccine (Measles, Mumps, Rubella): Usually given around 12-15 months of age. These three diseases can cause serious complications:

- Measles can cause pneumonia and brain inflammation
- Mumps can cause brain inflammation and deafness
- Rubella can cause serious birth defects if pregnant women get infected

Timing and Schedule Importance

Vaccines are given on specific schedules because this is when children need protection most. The schedule is designed to protect children before they're likely to be exposed to these diseases.

Some vaccines are given very early because babies are at highest risk for severe complications from certain diseases. Others are given later when the child's immune system is more mature and can respond better to the vaccine.

Missing vaccines or delaying them leaves children vulnerable during the time when they need protection most. It's important to follow the recommended schedule as closely as possible.

If a child misses vaccines due to illness or other circumstances, they can usually catch up. Healthcare providers can help determine the best schedule for catch-up vaccinations.

Vaccines for Specific Risks

In areas where certain diseases are common, additional vaccines may be recommended:

Yellow fever vaccine: In areas where yellow fever occurs, usually given around 9-12 months of age. - Yellow fever is a mosquito- borne viral disease characterized by fever, muscle pain, and sometimes severe liver damage leading to jaundice

Meningitis vaccines: May be recommended in areas where meningitis outbreaks occur - Meningitis is a serious inflammation of the membranes covering the brain and spinal cord, most common in babies. Symptoms in infants include fever, constant crying, poor feeding, extreme sleepiness or irritability, and a high-pitched cry. Other signs can be a tense, bulging soft spot (fontanelle) on the head, a stiff neck, or a rash that doesn't fade when pressed (use the glass test).

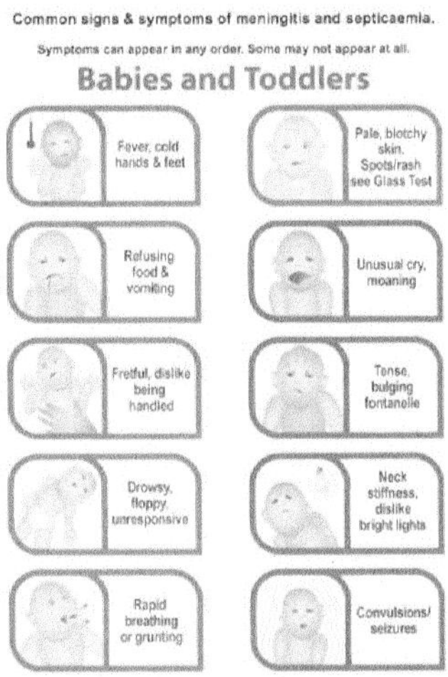

Pic 98: https://afuncan.com/#

Japanese encephalitis vaccine: In areas where this mosquito- borne disease is common. - **Acute Encephalitis Syndrome (AES)** is the clinical presentation of severe JE in children, characterized by rapid progression of symptoms including fever, severe headache, altered mental state, seizures, and coma. JE is a viral disease spread by mosquitoes, most common in children and causing severe neurological problems in severe cases.

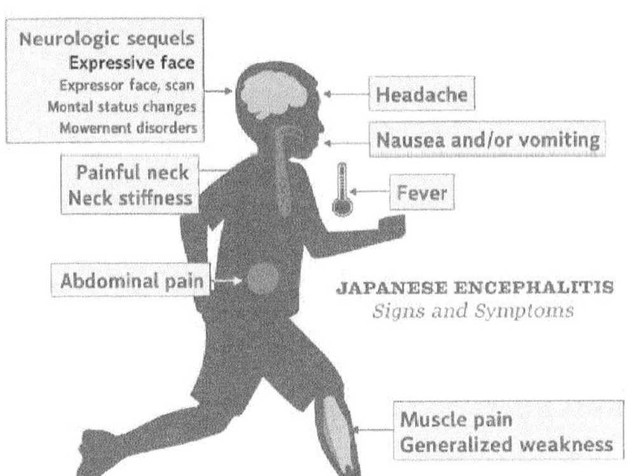

Pic 99: https://www.kauveryhospital.com/

Pic 99: https://www.kauveryhospital.com/

Rotavirus vaccine: Protects against severe diarrhea caused by rotavirus, usually given as drops by mouth.

Rotavirus in children typically leads to severe gastroenteritis, causing symptoms like watery diarrhea, vomiting, and fever, with the most significant risk being dehydration, which can be severe and even life-threatening. Other potential complications include lethargy, irritability, and, in rare cases, central nervous system issues such as encephalopathy. Treatment focuses on preventing and treating dehydration through fluid and electrolyte replacement.

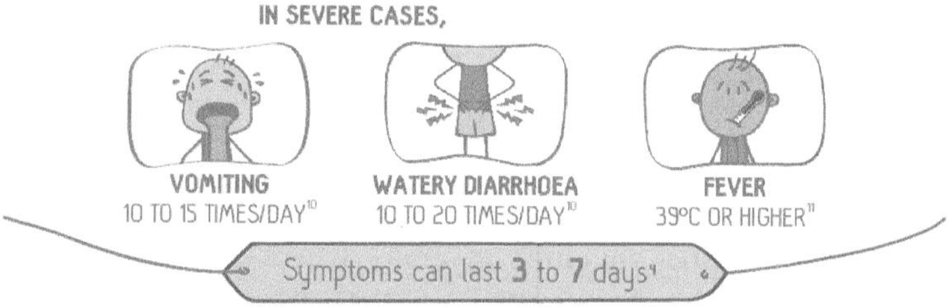

Pic 100: https://theprotectors.my/rotavirus-protectors

Addressing Common Vaccine Concerns with Facts

"Vaccines Cause Autism"

This concern has been thoroughly studied by scientists around the world. Large studies involving millions of children have found no link between vaccines and autism.

The original study that suggested this link was found to be fraudulent - the researcher made up data and lost his medical license. The medical journal that published the study took it back.

Autism is usually diagnosed around the same time children receive certain vaccines, which led some people to think vaccines caused autism. But this is like saying roosters cause the sun to rise because roosters crow before sunrise.

"Natural Immunity is Better"

While it's true that getting a disease naturally can provide strong immunity, this comes with serious risks. Natural infections can cause complications, permanent disability, or death.

Vaccines provide immunity without these risks. They train your immune system to recognize germs without exposing you to the full disease.

Some vaccine-prevented diseases are so serious that getting them naturally carries a high risk of death or permanent damage. Measles, for example, kills about 1-2 children out of every 1,000 who get it naturally.

"Too Many Vaccines at Once"

Children's immune systems are much stronger than many people realize. Every day, children are exposed to thousands of germs and their immune systems handle them easily.

The number of germs in vaccines is tiny compared to what children encounter naturally. Getting multiple vaccines at once is actually easier on the immune system than spreading them out over many visits.

Delaying vaccines leaves children vulnerable to dangerous diseases for longer periods. The recommended schedule protects children when they need it most.

"Vaccines Contain Dangerous Ingredients"

Vaccine ingredients are carefully tested for safety. The amounts of preservatives or other ingredients in vaccines are much smaller than what people encounter in food, water, and the environment every day.

For example, there is more formaldehyde in a single pear than in any vaccine. There is more aluminum in breast milk than in vaccines.

All vaccine ingredients serve important purposes - preserving the vaccine, helping it work better, or preventing contamination.

Fear of Side Effects

Most vaccine side effects are mild - soreness at the injection site, low fever, or fussiness for a day or two. These are signs that the immune system is responding to the vaccine.

Serious side effects from vaccines are extremely rare - much rarer than serious complications from the diseases vaccines prevent.

The risks of not vaccinating are much greater than the risks of vaccinating. For example, measles kills about 1,000 times more children than the measles vaccine causes serious problems.

Nutrition's Role in Children's Immunity

Adequate Calories for Growth

Children need enough calories not just to grow bigger, but to build and maintain their immune systems. Malnourished children get sick more often and have more serious complications from infections.

When children don't get enough food, their bodies focus on essential functions for survival and may not produce enough immune cells and antibodies to fight infections effectively.

Even mild malnutrition can weaken immune function. Children who seem to be growing normally but don't get enough vitamins and minerals may still have weak immune systems.

Protein for Immune Cell Production

Protein is especially important for immune function because immune cells and antibodies are made primarily of protein. Children who don't get enough protein cannot make enough infection-fighting cells.

Good protein sources include beans, lentils, eggs, meat, fish, dairy products, and nuts (for children old enough to eat them safely). Even small amounts of animal protein can significantly improve a child's immune function.

Combining different plant proteins (like rice and beans) can provide complete protein even when meat is not available or affordable.

Essential Vitamins and Minerals

Vitamin A: Important for maintaining barriers against infection (skin, lining of airways and digestive tract). Found in orange and yellow vegetables, dark leafy greens, and animal products.

Vitamin C: Helps immune cells work effectively. Found in citrus fruits, tomatoes, and many vegetables.

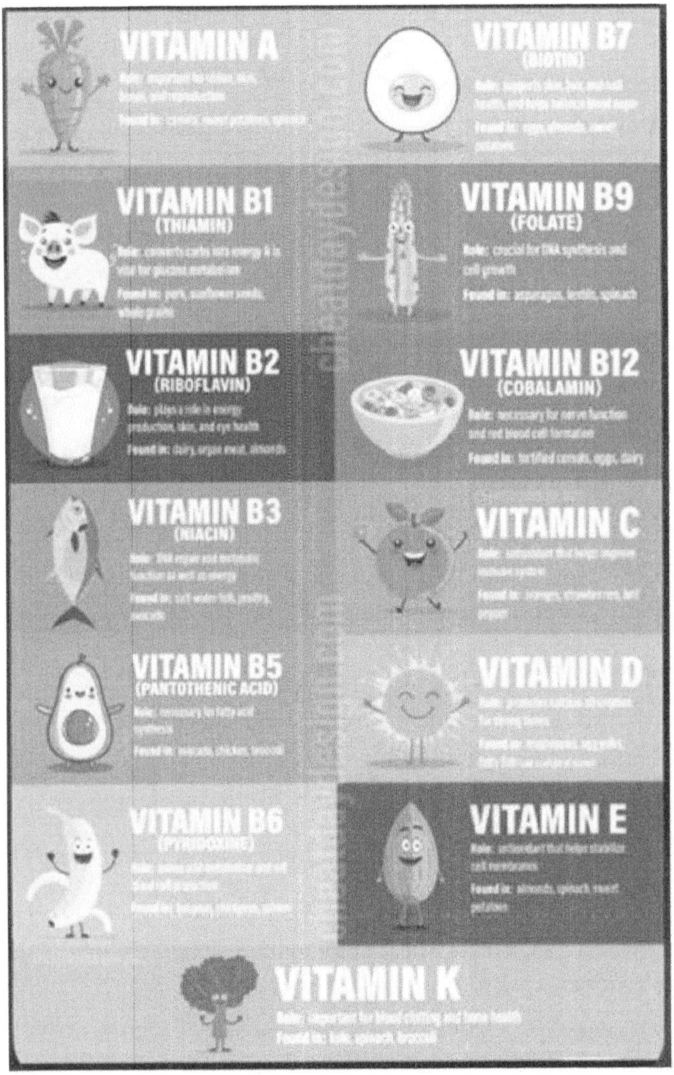

Pic 101: https://in.pinterest.com/pin/22532078761010543O/

Iron: Needed for immune cells to function properly. Found in meat, beans, leafy greens, and fortified foods.

Zinc: Essential for immune function. Found in meat, beans, nuts, and seeds.

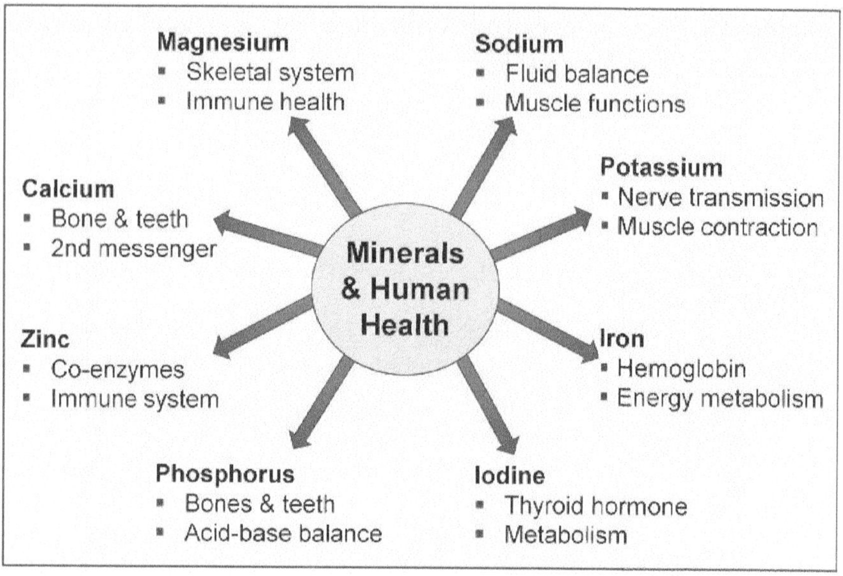

Pic 102: https://www.mdpi.com/2072-6643/17/3/454

Children who eat a variety of foods are more likely to get the nutrients they need for strong immune systems.

Breastfeeding Benefits

Breast milk provides antibodies from the mother that help protect babies from infections during their first months of life. These antibodies are especially important before babies can be fully vaccinated.

Breastfeeding also helps establish healthy bacteria in the baby's digestive system, which supports immune function throughout life.

Even in areas where clean water is available, breast milk is usually safer and more nutritious than formula for babies.

Community Focus: Accessing Vaccination Programs

Finding Vaccination Services

Government health centers: Most countries have government vaccination programs that provide vaccines free or at low cost. These are usually the most reliable source of vaccines.

Community health workers: Trained community health workers may provide certain vaccines, especially during vaccination campaigns.

NGO programs: Non-governmental organizations may provide vaccination services, especially during emergencies or in underserved areas.

Mobile vaccination teams: Some programs bring vaccines directly to communities using mobile teams that visit on specific dates.

Religious or community centers: These may serve as vaccination sites during campaigns or regular programs.

Vaccination Campaigns

Mass vaccination campaigns target specific diseases or age groups. These campaigns may vaccinate all children in a community over a few days or weeks.

Campaign vaccines are usually safe and effective, even if given outside of regular healthcare facilities. The vaccines are the same ones used in regular programs.

During campaigns, it's important to bring any vaccination records you have so health workers know what vaccines your child has already received.

Even if your child has been vaccinated before, they may need additional doses of certain vaccines during campaigns.

Maintaining Vaccine Schedules

Keep vaccination records: Maintain a record of all vaccines your child has received, including dates. This helps ensure they get all needed vaccines and don't get unnecessary repeats.

Regular check-ups: If possible, take children for regular health check-ups where vaccination status can be reviewed and missing vaccines identified.

Make-up appointments: If your child misses a scheduled vaccine due to illness or other circumstances, schedule a make-up appointment as soon as possible.

Travel considerations: If you plan to travel with children, check if they need additional vaccines for the areas you'll visit.

VACCINES FOR THE FIRST YEAR OF BIRTH

CONSULT WITH YOUR DOCTOR FIRST !

THIS LIST IS A COMBINATION OF IAP AND UIP VACCINES

Age	Vaccine	Disease	Dose
Birth	BCG	Tuberculosis	Only dose
	OPV	Polio	1st Dose
	Hep B	Hepatitis B	1st Dose
6 Weeks	OPV	Polio	2nd Dose
	IPV/ OPV	Polio	1st Dose
	Hep B (Pentavac Vaccine*)	Hepatitis B	2nd Dose
	DPTw (Pentavac Vaccine*)	Diphtheria, Whooping cough, Tetanus	1st Dose
	Hib (Pentavac Vaccine*)	*Haemophilus influenzae* type b	1st Dose
	Rotavirus**	Rotavirus	1st Dose
	Pneumococcal Vaccine	Pneumonia, Meningitis, Sepsis	1st Dose
10 Weeks	DPTw	Diphtheria, Whooping cough, Tetanus	2nd Dose
	IPV / OPV	Polio	2nd Dose
	Hib	*Haemophilus influenzae* type b	2nd Dose
	Rotavirus**	Rotavirus	2nd Dose
	Pneumococcal Vaccine	Pneumonia, Meningitis, Sepsis	2nd Dose
14 Weeks	DPTw	Diphtheria, Whooping cough, Tetanus	3rd Dose
	IPV / OPV	Polio	3rd Dose
	Hib	*Haemophilus influenzae* type b	3rd Dose
	Rotavirus**	Rotavirus	3rd Dose
	Pneumococcal Vaccine	Pneumonia, Meningitis, Sepsis	3rd Dose
6 Months	OPV	Polio	4th Dose
	Hep B	Hepatitis B	3rd Dose (at 24 weeks & at least 16 weeks after the first dose)
9 Months	OPV	Polio	5th Dose
	MMR	Measles, Mumps ,Rubella	1st Dose
9- 12 Months	Typhoid conjugate vaccine	Typhoid	4 weeks after the measles vaccine
12 Months	Hep A 1**	Hepatitis A	1st/Only Dose

● Highlighted vaccines are UIP vaccines prescribed as mandatory by the govenment.

** There are different types of vaccines. Please check with your doctor.

WPA whatparentsask.com

VACCINES FOR THE SECOND YEAR OF BIRTH

CONSULT WITH YOUR DOCTOR FIRST !

THIS LIST IS A COMBINATION OF IAP AND UIP VACCINES

Age	Vaccine	Disease	Dose
15 Months	MMR	Measles, Mumps ,Rubella	2nd dose in 2nd Year
	Varicella	Chickenpox	1st dose after 15 months
	Pneumococcal Vaccine	Pneumonia, Meningitis , Sepsis	Booster
16 Months	DPTw	Diphtheria, Whooping cough, Tetanus	Booster
	IPV	Polio	Booster
	Hib	*Haemophilus influenzae* type b	Booster
18 Months	Hep A	Hepatitis A *	This dose depends on which vaccine was taken the first time.
2 Years	Typhoid Vaccine	Typhoid	Depends on which vaccine was taken the first time
4- 6 Years	DPTw	Diphtheria, Whooping cough, Tetanus	Booster
	OPV	Polio	Booster
	Varicella	Chickenpox	2nd dose 3 months after 1st dose
	MMR	Measles, Mumps ,Rubella	Booster
10 -12 Years	Td / Tdap	Tetanus,Diptheria	Tdap is preferred every 10 years
	HPV	Human Papilloma virus	1st Dose

● Highlighted vaccines are UIP vaccines prescribed as mandatory by the govenment.

* There are different types of vaccines. Please check with your doctor.

WPA® whatparentsask.com

Pic 103: https://whatparentsask.com/vaccination-chart- india-commonly-asked-questions/

Overcoming Barriers to Vaccination

Transportation: If vaccination sites are far away, organize with other families to share transportation costs or arrange group visits.

Work schedules: Some vaccination programs offer services on weekends or evenings to accommodate working parents.

Cost concerns: Many vaccination programs are free or low-cost. Ask about financial assistance if cost is a barrier.

Cultural concerns: Discuss any cultural or religious concerns with healthcare providers, who can often address these while still providing protection for your child.

Language barriers: Bring someone who can translate if needed, or ask if interpreters are available.

Chapter - 10
Prevention is the Best Medicine

"Stopping infections before they start"

Hand Hygiene and When It Matters Most

Why Hand Washing Works

Your hands touch hundreds of surfaces every day that may have germs on them. These germs can live on your hands for hours, waiting for the chance to enter your body through your mouth, nose, or eyes.

Hand washing with soap physically removes germs from your hands and washes them away. It doesn't just kill germs - it removes them completely so they can't infect you.

Even plain water helps remove some germs, but soap is much more effective. Soap breaks down the protective layers around many germs and helps wash them away more completely.

Proper Hand Washing Technique

Use soap and clean water: Any soap works - it doesn't have to be antibacterial soap. The scrubbing action and soap are what remove germs.

Scrub all surfaces: Wash palms, backs of hands, between fingers, under fingernails, and around wrists. Many people miss the areas between fingers and under fingernails.

Scrub for 20 seconds: This is about the time it takes to sing "Happy Birthday" twice. Counting to 20 slowly also works.

Rinse thoroughly: Use clean running water to rinse away all soap and loosened germs.

Dry with a clean towel or air dry: Clean hands can get contaminated again from dirty towels.

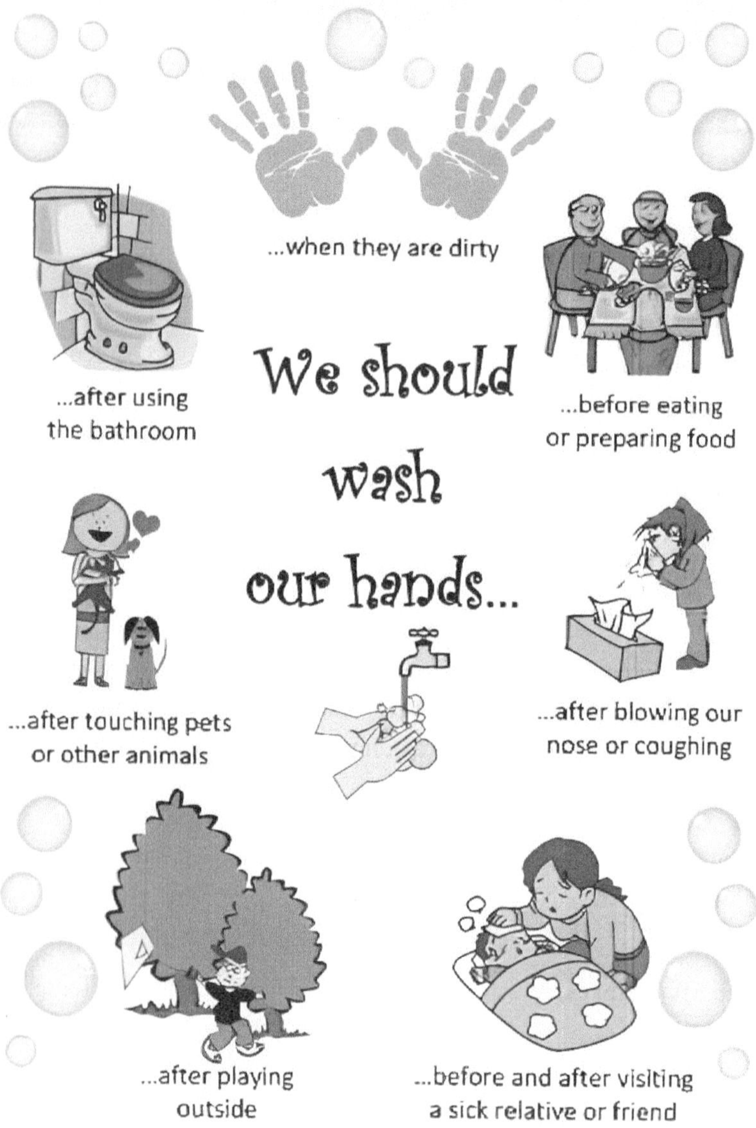
We should wash our hands...
...when they are dirty
...after using the bathroom
...before eating or preparing food
...after touching pets or other animals
...after blowing our nose or coughing
...after playing outside
...before and after visiting a sick relative or friend

Pic 104: https://in.pinterest.com/pin/884605551785338759/ When Hand Washing is Most Important

Before eating or preparing food: This prevents germs on your hands from getting into your mouth or contaminating food.

After using the toilet: Human waste contains many germs that can cause serious illness.

After coughing, sneezing, or blowing your nose: This prevents spreading germs to other people and surfaces.

After touching animals or animal waste: Animals can carry germs that make humans sick.

After handling garbage or dirty objects: These can contaminate your hands with various germs.

Before and after caring for sick people: This protects both you and the sick person.

After touching shared surfaces: Doorknobs, handrails, and other surfaces touched by many people can harbor germs.

Alternatives When Soap and Water Aren't Available-

Alcohol-based hand sanitizer: Should contain at least 60% alcohol to be effective. Use enough to cover all hand surfaces and rub until dry.

Clean sand or ash: In emergency situations, rubbing hands vigorously with clean sand or ash can help remove some germs.

Clean cloth: Wiping hands thoroughly with a clean, dry cloth removes some germs through friction.

Remember that these alternatives are not as effective as soap and water, but they're better than nothing when proper hand washing isn't possible.

Safe Food and Water Practices Water Safety

Boiling water: Brings water to a rolling boil for at least one minute to kill most germs. Let it cool before drinking. This is the most reliable method when you're unsure about water safety.

Water storage: Store treated water in clean, covered containers. Don't put your hands or dirty utensils into stored water.

Source protection: Use the cleanest water source available. Flowing water is usually safer than stagnant water.

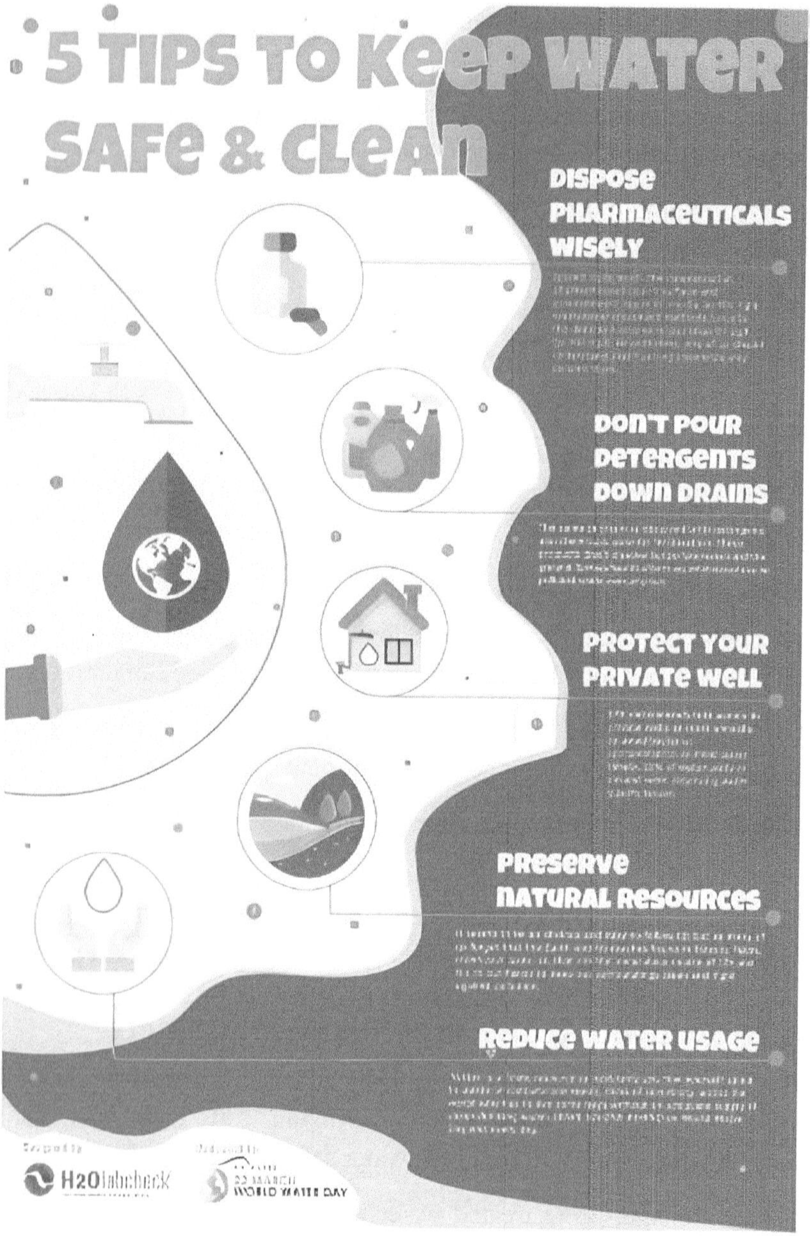
5 TIPS TO KEEP WATER SAFE & CLEAN
DISPOSE PHARMACEUTICALS WISELY
DON'T POUR DETERGENTS DOWN DRAINS
PROTECT YOUR PRIVATE WELL
PRESERVE NATURAL RESOURCES
REDUCE WATER USAGE
H2Olabcheck
22 MARCH
WORLD WATER DAY

Pic 105: https://www.h2olabcheck.com/blog/view/5-tips- to-keep-water-clean-and-safe-on-world-water-day

Treatment options: If boiling isn't possible, water purification tablets or household bleach (2 drops per liter) can help disinfect water.

Food Safety Principles

Cook food thoroughly: Heat kills most germs. Cook meat until it's no longer pink inside, and make sure eggs are cooked until both yolk and white are firm.

Eat food while it's hot: Germs multiply rapidly in warm food. Eat cooked food soon after cooking, while it's still hot.

Avoid risky foods: Raw or undercooked meat, eggs, and seafood carry higher risk of germs. Unpasteurized dairy products can also be risky.

Choose safer street food: If buying prepared food, choose vendors who cook food fresh and serve it hot. Avoid foods that have been sitting at room temperature.

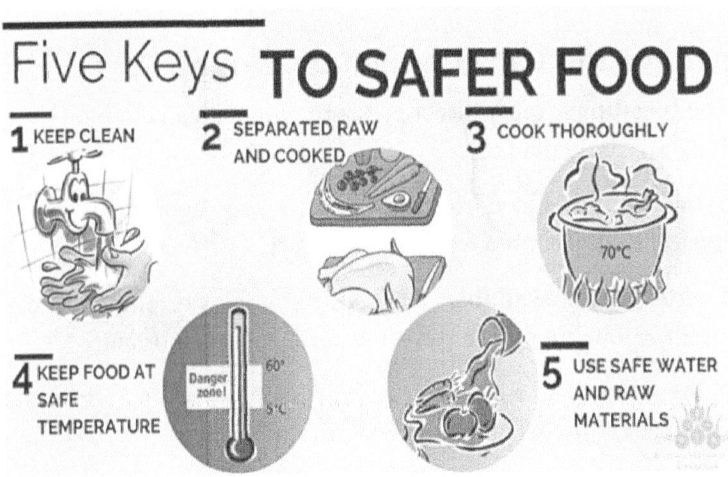
Five Keys TO SAFER FOOD
1 KEEP CLEAN
2 SEPARATED RAW AND COOKED
3 COOK THOROUGHLY
70°C
4 KEEP FOOD AT SAFE TEMPERATURE
Danger zone!
60°
5°C
5 USE SAFE WATER AND RAW MATERIALS

Pic 106: https://www.chshb.gov.tw/en/node/569#gsc.tab=0

Food Preparation Safety

Clean preparation surfaces: Wash cutting boards, knives, and counters with soap and water before preparing food.

Separate raw and cooked foods: Use different cutting boards and utensils for raw meat and other foods, or wash them thoroughly between uses.

Wash fruits and vegetables: Even if you plan to peel them, wash fruits and vegetables with clean water before eating or cooking.

Keep hot foods hot and cold foods cold: Don't leave cooked food at room temperature for more than 2 hours.

Food Storage without Refrigeration

Use food quickly: In hot climates, cooked food should be eaten within a few hours of cooking.

Keep food covered: Protect food from flies and other insects that can carry germs.

Store dry foods properly: Keep grains, beans, and other dry foods in sealed containers away from moisture and pests.

Preserve food safely: Traditional preservation methods like drying, salting, or smoking can make food safer when done properly.

Proper Wound Care Immediate Wound Care

Stop the bleeding: Apply direct pressure with a clean cloth or your hand if nothing else is available.

Clean the wound: Once bleeding stops, clean the wound gently with clean water. Remove any visible dirt or debris.

Apply antiseptic if available: Antiseptic solutions or ointments can help prevent infection, but cleaning with water is most important.

Cover the wound: Use a clean bandage, cloth, or even a clean piece of clothing to cover the wound and keep dirt out.

Ongoing Wound Care

Keep the wound clean and dry: Change bandages daily or when they become dirty or wet.

Watch for signs of infection: Increasing redness, swelling, warmth, pus, or red streaks extending from the wound.

Allow air circulation: Once the wound starts healing, remove bandages for short periods to let air reach the wound.

Don't pick at scabs: Let the natural healing process occur without interference.

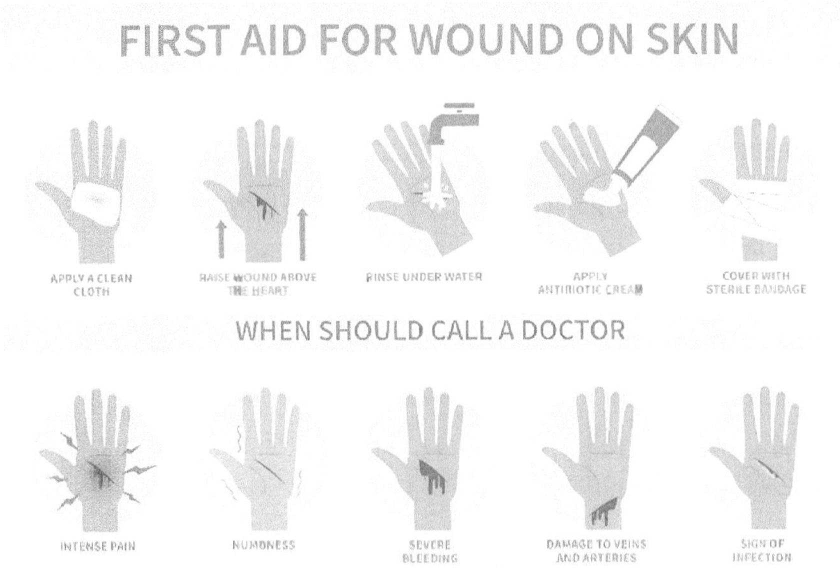

Pic 107: https://www.shutterstock.com/

When to Seek Help for Wounds

Deep cuts: Wounds that you can't clean thoroughly or that gape open may need stitches.

Puncture wounds: Deep wounds from nails, thorns, or other objects have high infection risk.

Animal bites: These carry high risk of infection and may need special treatment.

Signs of infection: Any wound that becomes more red, swollen, or painful after the first day or two.

Tetanus concerns: If you haven't had a tetanus vaccination recently and the wound was caused by a dirty or rusty object.

Environmental Cleanliness in Limited-Resource Settings Home Environment

Adequate ventilation: Open windows and doors when possible to allow fresh air circulation and reduce concentration of airborne germs.

Reduce overcrowding: When possible, arrange sleeping and living spaces to reduce the number of people breathing the same air.

Clean surfaces regularly: Wipe down frequently touched surfaces like tables, doorknobs, and light switches with soap and water.

Manage humidity: In very humid conditions, try to keep living areas as dry as possible to prevent mold and bacteria growth.

Waste Management

Human waste: Use proper toilet facilities when available. If not available, bury human waste at least 200 feet from water sources and living areas.

Garbage disposal: Remove garbage regularly from living areas. Compost organic waste if possible, or dispose of it away from the home.

Recycling: Containers that held food or drink should be cleaned before reuse to prevent contamination.

Animal waste: Keep animal waste away from living areas, food preparation areas, and water sources.

Water and Drainage

Eliminate standing water: Remove or cover containers that collect rainwater, which can become breeding sites for mosquitoes.

Improve drainage: Direct water away from living areas to prevent puddles and mud that can harbor germs.

Protect water sources: Keep toilets, garbage, and animal areas away from wells, springs, and other water sources.

Clean water containers: Regularly wash and dry containers used for storing drinking water.

Pest Control

Food storage: Keep food in sealed containers to prevent attracting rodents and insects.

Remove attractants: Clean up food crumbs and spills promptly to avoid attracting pests.

Block entry points: Seal cracks and holes where rodents and insects can enter homes.

Natural deterrents: Some plants and herbs can help repel insects naturally.

Community Focus: Community-Based Prevention Strategies

Collective Hygiene Efforts

Community clean-up days: Organize regular community efforts to clean shared spaces, remove garbage, and eliminate mosquito breeding sites.

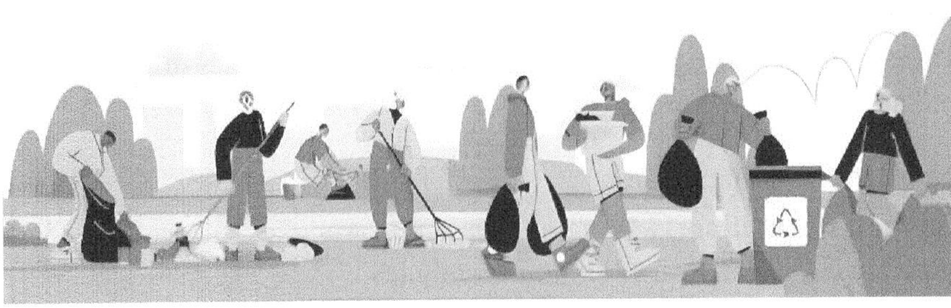

Pic 108: https://www.vecteezy.com/

Shared facility maintenance: Work together to maintain shared toilets, water sources, and washing areas in good condition.

Education programs: Share knowledge about hygiene and disease prevention throughout the community.

Resource sharing: Pool resources to purchase soap, cleaning supplies, or other hygiene materials in bulk.

Water and Sanitation Improvements

Community water treatment: Organize group efforts to treat and store water safely for community use.

Toilet construction: Work together to build and maintain adequate toilet facilities for the community.

Drainage projects: Undertake community projects to improve drainage and prevent standing water.

Well protection: Protect community water sources from contamination through collective action.

Disease Prevention Networks

Early warning systems: Develop community networks to quickly identify and report disease outbreaks.

Isolation support: Help families isolate sick members by providing food, water, and other necessities.

Vaccination promotion: Encourage and facilitate vaccination programs for all community members.

Information sharing: Ensure health information reaches all community members, including those who may be isolated or marginalized.

Emergency Preparedness

Supply stockpiling: Maintain community supplies of basic medical materials, soap, and water treatment supplies.

Emergency communication: Develop systems for communicating health emergencies to authorities and within the community.

Mutual aid agreements: Arrange for communities to help each other during health emergencies or outbreaks.

Training programs: Train community members in basic first aid and disease prevention techniques.

Chapter - 11
Home Remedies and When to Use Them

"Traditional wisdom meets modern knowledge"

Effective Home Treatments

Hydration - The Foundation of Home Care

Water is the most important home remedy for most illnesses. When you're sick, your body needs extra fluids to replace what's lost through fever, sweating, vomiting, or diarrhea.

For fever: Drinking plenty of fluids helps prevent dehydration and may help bring down fever. Cool water is best, but any clean fluid helps.

For respiratory infections: Fluids help thin mucus, making it easier to cough up. Warm liquids like teas or broths can be especially soothing.

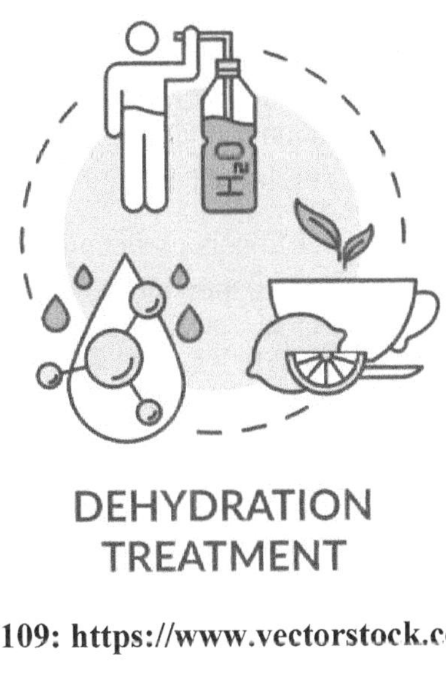

Pic 109: https://www.vectorstock.com/

For digestive illnesses: Small, frequent sips of clear fluids help prevent dehydration when you can't keep large amounts down.

Oral rehydration solution: Mix 1 teaspoon of salt and 2 tablespoons of sugar in 1 liter of clean water. This helps replace essential minerals lost during diarrhea and vomiting.

Rest - Letting Your Body Heal

Rest is one of the most powerful home remedies, yet it's often overlooked. When you rest, your body can focus energy on fighting infection instead of on daily activities.

Sleep: Your body produces more infection-fighting cells during sleep. Try to sleep more than usual when you're sick.

Physical rest: Avoid strenuous activities that use energy your body needs for healing.

Mental rest: Stress can weaken your immune system, so try to reduce worries and mental strain while recovering.

Creating rest conditions: Make the sleeping area as comfortable as possible - cool, quiet, and dark.

Steam and Heat Therapy

Steam inhalation: Breathing steam from hot water can help relieve congestion and soothe irritated airways. Be careful to avoid burns from hot water or steam.

Warm compress: A warm, damp cloth applied to the forehead or chest can provide comfort during respiratory infections.

Humidified air: Hanging wet towels in sleeping areas or placing bowls of water near the bed can help add moisture to dry air.

Warm baths: If possible, warm baths can help reduce fever and provide comfort, but avoid them if the person is very weak or has certain conditions.

Traditional Herbal Remedies with Evidence

Ginger: Can help reduce nausea and may have anti-inflammatory properties. Can be made into tea or chewed fresh.

Honey: Has antibacterial properties and can soothe sore throats. Don't give honey to babies under 1 year old.

Garlic: Has antimicrobial properties and may help boost immune function. Can be eaten raw or cooked.

Turmeric: Has anti-inflammatory properties. Can be mixed with warm milk or used in cooking.

Lemon: Provides vitamin C and can help with hydration when added to water.

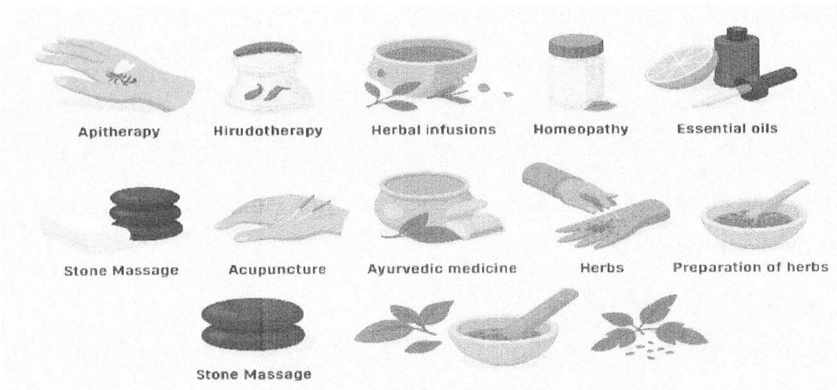

Pic 110: https://www.freepik.com/

Dangerous Home Remedies to Avoid Remedies That Can Cause Harm

Alcohol for fever: Rubbing alcohol on the skin to reduce fever can cause dangerous drops in body temperature and alcohol poisoning through skin absorption.

Ice baths for fever: Extreme cold can cause shivering, which actually raises body temperature and can be dangerous.

Aspirin for children: Can cause a serious condition called Reye's syndrome in children with viral infections.

Unpasteurized animal products: Raw milk, blood, or other animal products can contain dangerous bacteria and parasites.

Unknown plants or herbs: Many plants are poisonous, and some traditional remedies from one area may be dangerous if the wrong plant is used.

Potentially Harmful Practices

Forcing fluids during vomiting: If someone is actively vomiting, forcing them to drink can cause choking. Give small sips when vomiting stops.

Restricting food during fever: The body needs nutrients to fight infection. Offer nutritious foods that the person can tolerate.

Excessive heat application: Very hot compresses or heating pads can cause burns, especially when someone is too sick to move away from heat.

Delaying medical care: Some home remedies can provide comfort but shouldn't delay proper medical treatment for serious conditions.

Unsafe Herbal Preparations

Unknown dosages: Traditional medicines may be safe in small amounts but dangerous in large quantities.

Contaminated preparations: Herbal medicines made in unsanitary conditions can introduce additional infections.

Drug interactions: Some herbal remedies can interact dangerously with modern medicines.

Allergic reactions: Even natural remedies can cause allergic reactions in some people.

Supporting the Body's Healing Process Nutrition During Illness

Easy-to-digest foods: When appetite is poor, offer foods that are easy on the stomach like rice, bananas, or clear broths.

Small, frequent meals: Instead of large meals, offer small amounts of food more often to help maintain nutrition without overwhelming the digestive system.

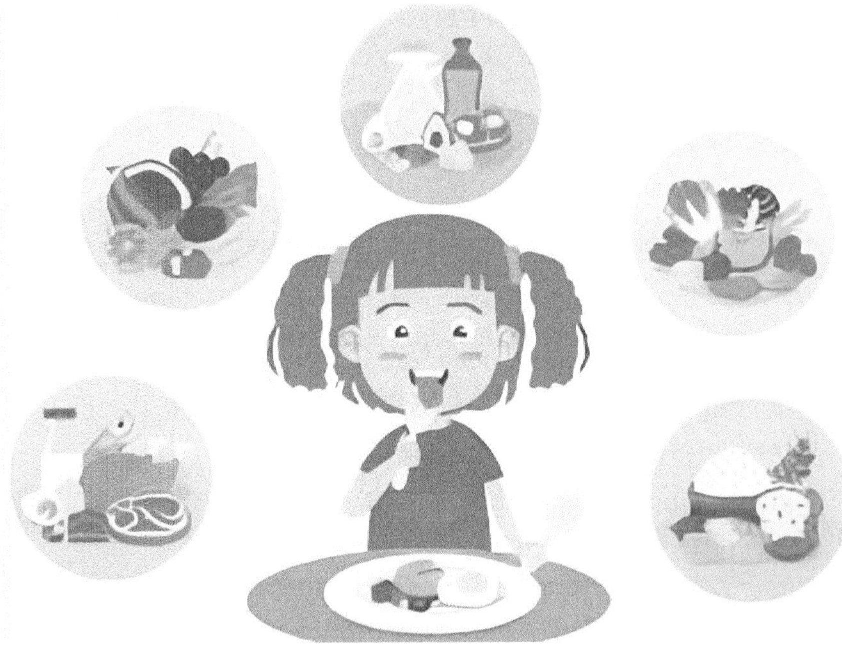

Pic 111: https://www.vecteezy.com/

Nutrient-rich options: When possible, include foods rich in vitamins and minerals that support immune function.

Foods to avoid: Very spicy, fatty, or hard-to-digest foods may worsen nausea or digestive symptoms.

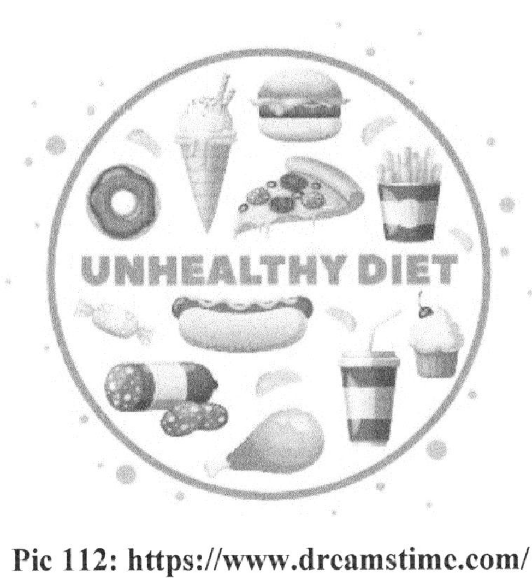

Pic 112: https://www.dreamstime.com/

Creating a Healing Environment

Comfortable temperature: Keep the sick person comfortable - not too hot or too cold.

Clean surroundings: Maintain cleanliness around the sick person to prevent additional infections.

Quiet space: Reduce noise and distractions to promote rest and recovery.

Fresh air: Ensure good ventilation while avoiding cold drafts.

Monitoring and Support

Track symptoms: Keep track of fever, appetite, fluid intake, and other symptoms to identify improvements or worsening.

Emotional support: Illness can be frightening, especially for children. Provide reassurance and comfort.

Gradual return to activity: As the person recovers, gradually increase activity levels rather than jumping back to normal routines immediately.

Prevent spread: Take measures to prevent the illness from spreading to other family members.

When to Combine Traditional and Modern Approaches Complementary Use of Home Remedies

Home remedies can often be used safely alongside modern medical treatments to provide additional comfort and support.

For symptom relief: Use home remedies to manage symptoms while modern medicine addresses the underlying cause of illness.

During recovery: Traditional supportive care can help speed recovery after medical treatment has begun.

For prevention: Many traditional practices for staying healthy can complement modern preventive measures.

Always inform healthcare providers: Tell medical professionals about any traditional remedies being used to avoid harmful interactions.

Recognizing Limitations

Home remedies for comfort only: Understand which traditional treatments provide comfort versus those claimed to cure serious diseases.

Time limits: Set reasonable time limits for trying home remedies before seeking modern medical care.

Severity guidelines: Know which symptoms require immediate medical attention regardless of traditional treatments.

Age considerations: Be especially cautious when using traditional remedies with very young children, elderly people, or pregnant women.

Integrating Approaches Safely

Start with proven home remedies: Use traditional treatments that have the best evidence for safety and effectiveness.

Monitor carefully: Watch for any signs that home remedies are causing harm or that the condition is worsening.

Seek guidance: When possible, consult with healthcare providers who understand both traditional and modern approaches.

Maintain open communication: Keep family members informed about all treatments being used.

Community Focus: Culturally Appropriate Healing Practices

Respecting Traditional Knowledge

Learning from elders: Older community members often have valuable knowledge about safe and effective traditional remedies.

Documenting practices: Record traditional practices that have proven safe and effective over generations.

Sharing responsibly: Share traditional knowledge while emphasizing safety and the importance of knowing when modern medical care is needed.

Preserving culture: Maintain cultural healing practices as part of community identity while ensuring safety.

Community Healing Resources

Traditional healers: Work with respected traditional healers who understand both the benefits and limitations of traditional medicine.

Medicinal plant cultivation: Grow and maintain traditional medicinal plants in community gardens or designated areas.

Knowledge exchange: Create opportunities for community members to share safe traditional practices.

Integration with modern care: Develop relationships between traditional healers and modern healthcare providers when possible.

Education and Safety

Safety first: Educate community members about which traditional practices are safe and which may be harmful.

Proper preparation: Ensure traditional medicines are prepared safely and hygienically.

Dosage guidelines: Establish community understanding of safe amounts and frequencies for traditional remedies.

Emergency protocols: Ensure everyone knows when to seek immediate modern medical care regardless of traditional treatments.

Building Bridges

Respectful dialogue: Encourage respectful communication between those who prefer traditional methods and those who favor modern medicine.

Best of both worlds: Help community members understand how traditional and modern approaches can work together for better health.

Training opportunities: Provide training on basic modern health practices while respecting traditional beliefs.

Community consensus: Work toward community agreement on when different types of healing approaches are most appropriate.

Chapter 12

Building Healthy Communities Working Together for Health

Community Hygiene and Sanitation

Healthy communities start with safe water, proper waste management, and clean public spaces. Shared water sources like wells and springs must be protected from human and animal waste, maintained regularly, and used responsibly to avoid contamination. Communities should establish rules for water use, train members to recognize signs of contamination, and act quickly when problems arise. Waste management requires safe toilets, organized garbage collection, recycling, composting, and proper drainage to prevent flooding and stagnant water. Public spaces such as markets, schools, religious centers, and transport areas should follow hygiene standards, while regular clean-up days, mosquito and vector control, and road maintenance keep the environment safe.

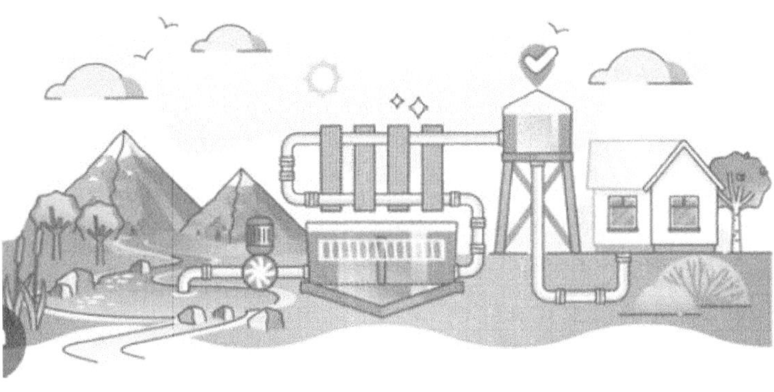

Pic 113: https://www.shutterstock.com/

Protecting Vulnerable Members

Children need safe play areas, school health programs, and systems that support families during illness, along with community safeguards against abuse. Elderly members benefit from regular check-ins, nutritional and medication support, and rapid emergency assistance. For people with disabilities, accessibility to toilets, water, and health centers is essential, alongside inclusion in education, vaccination, and emergency planning. During illness, communities can help families isolate patients, provide transport to health centers, share information, and offer economic support to households losing income.

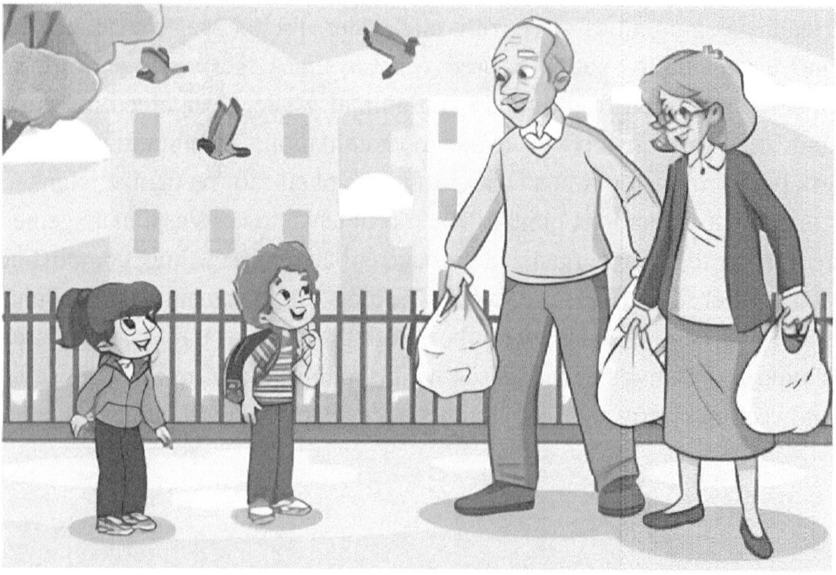

Pic 114: https://www.vecteezy.com/

Recognizing and Reporting Outbreaks

Communities play a crucial role in detecting and reporting unusual illness patterns, severe cases, or unexpected deaths. Certain diseases like measles, meningitis, and cholera require immediate reporting. Training community health workers, establishing information networks, and keeping illness records help track outbreaks. Quick response systems, coordination with authorities, and mobilizing resources allow effective control, while accurate reporting, rumor control, and respectful information sharing prevent panic and protect privacy.

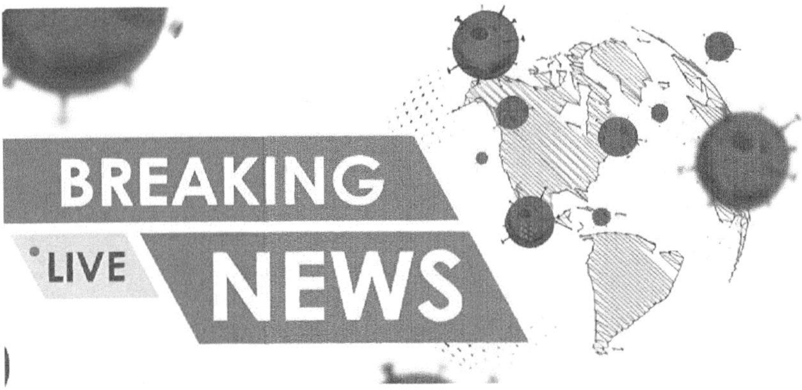

Pic 115: https://www.shutterstock.com/

Accessing Healthcare Resources

Strong communities know how to navigate healthcare services. This includes awareness of government facilities, private options, NGO programs, and traditional healers. Trained guides can assist with navigating systems, documentation, transportation, and language support. Communities can reduce financial barriers through health funds, resource sharing, and identifying free or low-cost services, while also providing emergency medical assistance. Education about patient rights, monitoring quality of care, and addressing discrimination ensures fair and equal access for all.

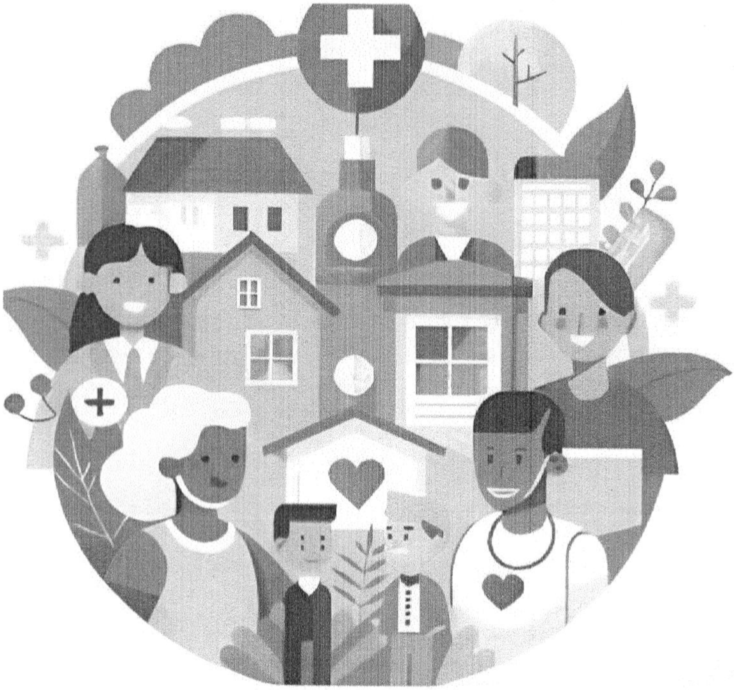

Pic 116: https://www.freepik.com/

Community Focus: Collective Action for Health Improvement

Sustainable health improvements depend on collective organization and leadership. Communities can form health committees, train leaders, and hold regular meetings to discuss priorities. Fundraising, grant applications, volunteer efforts, and resource sharing strengthen projects, while partnerships with governments, NGOs, neighboring communities, and businesses broaden impact. Long-term planning, capacity building, monitoring, and knowledge sharing make programs sustainable. Finally, advocacy efforts—through policy engagement, documentation, networking, and local media—help communities secure lasting improvements in health and wellbeing.